CW00674438

INTERPRE
CLINICAL
LABORAT

INTERPRETATION OF CLINICAL CHEMISTRY LABORATORY DATA

C.G. FRASER
BSc, PhD, FAACB

Top Grade Biochemist,
Ninewells Hospital and Medical School,
Dundee, Scotland

Honorary Senior Lecturer in Biochemical Medicine,
University of Dundee

BLACKWELL SCIENTIFIC PUBLICATIONS
Oxford Edinburgh London
Boston Palo Alto Melbourne

© 1986 by
Blackwell Scientific Publications
Editorial offices:
Osney Mead, Oxford, OX2 OEL
8 John Street, London, WC1N 2ES
23 Ainslie Place, Edinburgh, EH3
    6AJ
52 Beacon Street, Boston
    Massachusetts 02108, USA
667 Lytton Avenue, Palo Alto
    California 94301, USA
107 Barry Street, Carlton
    Victoria 3053, Australia

All rights reserved. No part of this
publication may be reproduced,
stored in a retrieval system, or
transmitted, in any form or by any
means, electronic, mechanical,
photocopying, recording or
otherwise without the prior
permission of the copyright owner

First published 1986

Photoset by Enset (Photosetting),
Midsomer Norton, Bath, Avon
and printed and bound
by Billing and Sons Ltd.,
Worcester

DISTRIBUTORS

USA
  Blackwell Mosby Book
  Distributors
  11830 Westline Industrial Drive
  St Louis, Missouri 63141

Canada
  The C.V. Mosby Company,
  5240 Finch Avenue East,
  Scarborough, Ontario.

Australia
  Blackwell Scientific Publications
  (Australia) Pty Ltd
  107 Barry Street, Carlton,
  Victoria 3053

British Library
Cataloguing in Publication Data

Fraser, Callum G.
  Interpretation of clinical
  chemistry laboratory data.
  1. Medicine, Clinical—
  Laboratory manuals
  I. Title
  610'.28   RB37

  ISBN 0-632-01579-9

Contents

Preface

Modern clinical laboratories offer a wide range of analytical services and the results of many of the tests provided are reported in numerical format. While there are a number of excellent concise textbooks available which deal with the contribution of clinical chemistry tests to medical care, particularly concerning selection of appropriate tests and interpretation of results, there appears to be lack of a basic text dealing with both the more numerical aspects of interpretation of clinical chemistry laboratory data and the many factors, other than disease, that affect the results of clinical laboratory tests, particularly those performed in the clinical chemistry laboratory.

This book was written to fill this need and to provide an up-to-date but concise summary of basic information hitherto only very briefly discussed in most basic texts or unavailable except in papers, reviews and more complex specialist books. The book is designed for the use of medical students in the later years of their courses and for those preparing for examinations in clinical chemistry, chemical pathology, medical laboratory sciences and medical technology. It is hoped that current users of clinical laboratory services will also read this book.

The material is based upon formal and informal teaching provided to both medical students and students reading for the degree of Master of Science in Clinical Biochemistry of the Flinders University of South Australia, and for students enrolled in the Batchelor of Medical Science degree of the University of Dundee. The book is designed to be complementary to basic texts on the more clinical aspects of clinical chemistry, for example, *A Guide to Diagnostic*

Clinical Chemistry by Walmsley and White (1983, Blackwell Scientific Publications Ltd., Melbourne) and *Lecture Notes on Clinical Chemistry* by Whitby, Percy-Robb and Smith (1984, 3rd ed., Blackwell Scientific Publications Ltd., Oxford). Each chapter deals with a discrete subject and further reading material is documented. This book, like the former text noted above, has some examples taken from actual laboratory practice. The more complex mathematical and statistical aids to the interpretation of test results which are not widely used in current practice are not dealt with in this text.

Clinical chemistry is a complex subject with its own terminology, theories and concepts. The scope of the discipline is so wide that it is impossible for either user, future user, the medical student, or new entrant to the professions employed in clinical laboratories to master every aspect of the subject or, perhaps more importantly, to judge the depth to which basic knowledge should be acquired. An important role for any basic text is to provide a guide to students and trainees about the breadth of knowledge that should be accumulated.

This text does cover the material required to be taught early in medical courses, as detailed by the Education Committee of the International Federation of Clinical Chemistry (Fraser C.G., Zinder O., de Cediel N., Porter C.J., Schwartz M.K. and Worth H.G.J., Guidelines [1985] for teaching of clinical chemistry to medical students. *Journal of Clinical Chemistry and Clinical Biochemistry* **23**, 697). It is hoped that it will, therefore, provide guidance to educators regarding the topics which should be taught in medical schools.

In preparing this text, Mr William A. Bartlett, Dr Lesley M. Nelson and Miss Catriona E.L. Boyle read all of the draft text and made many excellent suggestions. Miss Margaret C.K. Browning was a constant source of advice and encouragement. Mrs Margaret Cooper is sincerely thanked for typing all of the manuscript. Miss Maureen Sneddon of the Department of Medical Illustration very kindly drew all of the Figures and the cover illustration.

The author is of course responsible for all errors and omissions and would be grateful for suggestions and critical comment.

Callum G. Fraser
Department of Biochemical Medicine,
Ninewells Hospital and Medical School,
Dundee.
November 1985

Chapter 1
The Role of the
Clinical Chemistry Laboratory

1.1 Introduction

Many millions of clinical laboratory tests are performed each year throughout the world. In addition, the number of tests done continues to rise each year and, although there are a number of reasons for this ever increasing use of tests, many would suggest that there is little evidence that clinical care has improved in parallel.

There is little doubt that many clinical laboratory tests are requested without objective prior thought and therefore, in this first chapter, the use of the clinical chemistry laboratory will be discussed in detail. In addition, the consequences of the various possible approaches to the use of the clinical laboratory will be considered.

Interpretation of test results, particularly those of a numerical nature, is not always performed in the most rational manner and the influence of test requesting on interpretation will be discussed. In addition, the many other real and potential sources of difficulty, the main subject matter of this text, will be enumerated.

1.2 The increasing use of the clinical laboratory

The number of tests performed is, as mentioned earlier, increasing each year. There are many reasons why this trend continues, including the following (*see* Further reading[1]):

(i) Clinician factors

Increased scientific training of medical students
Increased reliance on test results
Investigation based on adherence to protocols
Unnecessary repetition of tests
Laboratory data overload
Misunderstanding of test results

(ii) Laboratory and scientific factors

Advent of multi-channel analytical equipment
Introduction of new tests
Failure to eliminate old unnecessary tests
Delays in reporting test results
New diagnostic and management strategies

(iii) Hospital factors

Introduction of new specialist units
Increased turnover of patients
Treatment of more severely ill patients
Changing spectrum of disease

(iv) Other factors

Danger of medical litigation
Growing public awareness of laboratory tests
Health care seen by the public as a right

Many articles and editorials in medical journals, unfortunately mainly of a very subjective nature, have stated that a significant proportion of clinical chemistry tests requested are unnecessary for optimal patient care. As a result, a body of literature exists which suggests that strong efforts must be made to reduce the number of clinical laboratory test requests of this type. In spite of the ostensible wide interest in this topic, there have been only a small number of objective studies on methods to bring about a reduction in clinical chemistry laboratory workload. It has been shown that positive strategies such as (i) feeding back the costs of tests to clinicians, (ii) placing clinicians in league tables according to their requesting habits and (iii) offering small financial incentives have no effect. In contrast, (i) limiting the number of tests that each clinician can request, (ii) intensive education on the uses and abuses of a particular test and (iii) introduction of structured problem orientated request forms can eliminate some of the clinical laboratory tests thought to be performed for illogical reasons.

The concept that many clinical laboratory tests are requested for other purposes than clinical care has been discussed most amusingly by Hardison (*see* Further reading[3]) who lists the following 'excuses' for such test requests:

the 'to be complete' excuse
the 'they say . . .' excuse
the 'we'll get into trouble if we don't' excuse
the 'if you don't order everything at once, it won't get done' excuse
the 'as long as he is in hospital, we might as well' excuse
the 'academic' excuse
the 'malpractice' excuse
the 'protocol' excuse
the 'if it were my mother or father, I'd want it done' excuse
the 'how do we know he doesn't have it?' excuse.

However, it is believed that it is inappropriate to suggest that most clinical laboratory tests are requested for these subjective reasons since there are many different clinical situations in which the results of clinical chemistry tests are vital to patient care.

1.3   Uses of clinical laboratory test results

Clinical chemistry test results are used for a variety of clinical purposes, including the following (*see* Further reading[6]):

Diagnosis

To make a diagnosis which cannot be established without performing the test. To substantiate a diagnosis which has been made on other grounds. To clarify problems in differential diagnosis.

Management

To determine whether complications have occurred. To assess the possible severity of the disease and the prognosis. To monitor the course of the disease and/or the success or otherwise of the therapy. To assess, by analysis of therapeutic drugs, whether the drug regime is being adhered to by the patient. To predict the response to medical or surgical treatment.

Screening

To detect disease in selected groups of the apparently healthy by use of specific tests. To apply a battery of tests to persons who are not patients seeking medical care. To apply generally a battery of tests to all patients (profiling).

Other uses

To assist in various aspects of clinical and laboratory research and development. To aid in a range of educational activities.

1.4 Diagnosis

In most cases, clinical laboratory tests performed on clinically ill patients are carried out to confirm either clinical suspicion or a more positive diagnosis. Indeed, it has been estimated by Young (*see* Further reading[9]) that about 75% of diagnoses are made on consideration of the history of the patient and a further 10–15% are made as a result of the physical examination. The number of diagnoses made solely as a consequence of clinical chemistry laboratory test results is, therefore, very small.

When test results are requested for diagnostic purposes, the following points must be borne in mind.

Few clinical laboratory tests are so specific that the results provide a definitive diagnosis.

Most assays are performed on specimens of serum or plasma and, for many constituents, the levels in these easily obtained biological fluids do not always reflect the true content of either the cells or the body; notable examples are potassium, phosphate and iron.

Certain organs and systems, for example, the liver and the renal system, have considerable reserve capacity and some commonly used clinical laboratory test results may not show impairment of function until advanced disease is present.

As will be discussed in detail in Chapter 7 of this text, the predictive value of a clinical laboratory test result does increase as the prevalence of disease increases. As a consequence, the population on whom clinical laboratory tests are requested should include a high proportion of ill persons, carefully selected by clinical judgement prior to the test being performed.

In addition, many preanalytical and analytical factors affect clinical laboratory test results. These, the main subject of this text, do lead to interpretative difficulties. Careful selection of those tests not prone to problems of these types will minimize the difficulties.

It should not be assumed, however, that, simply because the diagnosis is clinically clear, no clinical laboratory test is required. In many clinical situations it is very worthwhile to obtain baseline test results in order to monitor effectively the effects of subsequent therapy, for example, on indices of thyrometabolic status.

1.5 Management

In hospital situations, most clinical chemistry laboratory tests are performed to assist in the management of patients.

Many of the caveats detailed earlier regarding the use of test results in diagnosis are relevant when results are used in management.

In addition, a number of other points should be considered, particularly the question of how often clinical laboratory tests should be requested. This can be decided most objectively by consideration of, firstly, the time scale over which significant changes are likely to be seen and, secondly, whether the test result reported, even if it has numerically changed significantly from the previous result (*see* Chapter 6), will cause a change in therapy.

In general terms, the more unusual the result of a clinical laboratory test, the more severe is the disease process, although, as stated earlier, the facts that (i) often results of analyses of serum or plasma do not reflect cellular or body content and (ii) some organs and systems have considerable reserve, does make it difficult to relate test results directly to either disease severity or prognosis.

Therapeutic drug monitoring, a relatively new development in clinical chemistry, is, with certain important qualifications, very helpful particularly when (i) there is a narrow margin between therapeutic and toxic levels, (ii) disease is likely to affect the metabolism of the drug by the individual patient and (iii) there may be problems of compliance.

1.6 Screening

Screening is a term that is used for a variety of efforts which are rather different and should be discussed separately (*see* Further reading[5]).

Targeted screening is designed to exclude or confirm a specific disease using one (or more) clinical laboratory tests. This screening is based upon the assumption that, using clinical laboratory test results, early or latent disease can be discovered. Treatment can then be initiated at this stage in the natural history of the disease process so that, at a relatively small cost, individuals do not develop severe disease which will incur high costs, both financial and social. Examples of successful screening programmes of this type are assessment of all neonates for the presence of high blood levels of phenylalanine or thyrotrophin (TSH) to detect phenyl-ketonuria and neonatal hypothyroidism respectively.

Multiphasic screening is the application of a battery of procedures to detect disease. When this is performed by clinical chemistry laboratories on either new admissions to hospital or on every occasion when one or more component tests of the battery is or are requested, the term *profiling* can be used.

When persons seek clinical help and clinical laboratory tests are performed in order to detect the presence of diseases which are not related to the presenting problem, the correct term to use is *case finding*.

Strictly speaking, the term screening should be reserved for the identification of unrecognized disease or defect and therefore is applied only to procedures applied to apparently well persons.

The principles that should apply to such screening programmes were enunciated over a decade and a half ago by Wilson and Junger (*see* Further reading[8]) and are as follows:

Each clinical condition sought should be an important problem.

There should be a therapeutic regime which is accepted for
the treatment of the disease detected.

Facilities must be available for both the diagnosis and
treatment of the disease.

There should be a suitable test.

The test considered suitable should be acceptable to the
population being screened.

The latent or early symptomatic stages in the disease
progress should be able to be recognized.

The natural history of the disease process should be
adequately understood.

There should be an agreed policy on the population to be
regarded as patients and treated.

The costs of the screening programme should be carefully
assessed.

The screening programme should not be conducted once
only but should be an ongoing process.

In addition, when clinical laboratory tests are used in
screening programmes, further criteria should be met and the
test should have the following attributes:

be a simple procedure to administer

be relatively cheap

be quick to perform

provide results that are easy to interpret

allow fulfilment of certain of the criteria detailed above

The criteria are very difficult to fulfil and, except for the
neonatal screening programmes which have been set up in
many parts of the world, it is unlikely that any clinical
chemistry laboratory test meets them.

1.7   Profiling

The term profiling can be applied to the strategy of performing
a battery of tests on (i) patients newly admitted to hospital, (ii)

all specimens submitted to the laboratory for one (or more) components of the battery, (iii) persons who represent for any reason to a clinician of any type (case finding) and (iv) to individuals who have not presented for medical care.

In these situations, some of the alleged advantages of the profiling approach that might be thought relevant include the following:

The process saves valuable time because all or most of the test results that might be required for the individual patient to aid in diagnosis are available early in the care of the patient.

The availability of the data would ensure that clinically relevant facts were not missed.

Undiagnosed disease processes which were latent or early in their progress would be detected and treatment subsequently initiated.

The findings on patients with clearcut diagnoses and straightforward management provide good educational material.

Tests can be performed more cheaply with fewer laboratory staff required.

Larger numbers of tests performed show the laboratory to be highly productive. This supposed increased productivity generates more profit for the laboratory staff and/or hospital in some countries and can be used to 'justify' the allocation of further staff, equipment and budgetary resources.

Reassurance of the individual who does not have disease but seeks medical advice (the 'worried well') can be performed by the finding of all of the clinical laboratory test results within reference values.

Many of the reasons for requesting tests quoted by Hardison that were noted earlier in this chapter have been used to justify profiling.

However, there are many disadvantages to profiling including:

The provision of numerical data not really required by the

clinician provides difficulties in that the receiver of the report has to dissect relevant data from the many results reported. Certain clinical chemistry laboratories attempt to help the clinician by flagging test results which are outside the reference limits and/or by flagging test results which are deemed to be clinically important. This approach has three disadvantages: (a) the clinician may merely scan reports to check for flagged test results and not interpret carefully all the test results either singly or in combination, (b) a test result within the reference interval may be of prime importance in making or excluding a diagnosis, monitoring therapy or assessing prognosis and (c) a test result within the reference interval may be a rare value for a particular individual according to the usual variation around the homeostatic setting point of that individual (*see* Chapter 6).

The tests that make up the profile are often selected on the basis that they are simple and relatively inexpensive to perform, particularly on multi-channel analytical instruments. Moreover, the test characteristics have usually been designed for diagnostic or management uses.

The profile often produces unexpected test results, particularly worrying being those outside the reference intervals. There are many reasons why such results occur (Chapter 8) including (a) the incomplete documentation of the patient's characteristics and subsequent interpretation without taking these into account (Chapter 2), (b) incorrect specimen collection and transport (Chapter 3), (c) analytical errors (Chapter 4), (d) use of incorrect reference intervals and lack of appreciation of the statistical nature of such intervals which results in the facts that 5% of healthy individuals are, by definition, outside the intervals and that as more tests are performed more results of this type will occur (Chapter 5) and (e) biological variability (Chapter 6). The unexpected 'abnormal' test result is often ignored as being due to laboratory error but, in some cases, a cause for the result is sought by embarking upon a series of further investigations which may uncover no new facts; this has been described aptly by Rang (*see* Further reading[4]) as the *Ulysses syndrome* because Ulysses travelled round the known world and had many adventures but ended his journey at the point of origin. There is little doubt that many resources are expended in following up such test results.

Studies on the use of profiling in the hospital situation have shown that hospital stay is generally not shortened by the early availability of clinical chemistry profile data.

Analysis of the meaning of the test results outside the reference intervals has been performed on a number of occasions in studies involving hospital patients, patients seen by general practitioners and healthy people and has demonstrated that many of these results were to be expected from the clinical state of the patient, only a small number of tests were 'diagnostic' and many test results were inexplicable. The study of Whitehead and Wooton (*see* Further reading[7]) showed, for example, that of the 100% of tests performed, 77% were not actually requested. Of these, 15.9% were 'abnormal' and this was made up of 28% that were unexpected, 9% that were 'diagnostic' and 62% that were unexplained.

It is noteworthy that those tests which give a supposed high yield of diagnostic information, including serum glucose, urate and iron, also give the highest number of test results which cannot be explained. Follow up of the unexplained results after five years showed that the finding of a test result outside the reference interval did not generally mean that the patient had latent or early disease.

The analytical equipment required to analyse specimens for a large number of analytes is expensive and sophisticated data handling systems are a fairly necessary adjunct.

On many occasions, test results are required as part of a series, for example, plasma glucose levels in specimens collected during an oral glucose loading test and serum enzyme activities following myocardial infarction. It is obviously not necessary to perform clinical chemistry profiles in such situations.

At the present time, there is no doubt that it is generally considered that profiling is not the ideal approach to the requesting or performance of clinical chemistry laboratory tests.

1.8 Discretionary approaches

The current view is that discretionary approaches to the requesting of clinical laboratory tests should be adopted. The patient on whom tests are requested should be assessed as an individual and necessary tests requested.

The trend to this approach is being facilitated by newer laboratory instruments which allow selection of appropriate tests from the large array possible (random access analysers), the advent of discrete analysis of various types which have high throughput, the move towards the performance of some clinical chemistry tests closer to the patient (Chapter 4) and the advent in some countries of legislation which allows reimbursement only for clinically relevant tests ('diagnosis related groups'). Many clinical laboratories which have large multi-channel laboratories have also moved away from profiling by reporting those test results which have been requested and other tests judged to be clinically relevant while suppressing all other information obtained.

Discretionary requesting does not necessarily mean that each and every test result desired must be specifically requested. A common and logical approach is that related tests may be requested as a group, sometimes called an organ panel or organ profile. Common examples are:
urea and electrolytes comprising sodium, potassium, chloride, bicarbonate, urea and/or creatinine,

liver function tests comprising proteins, albumin, alkaline
  phosphatase, bilirubins and alanine aminotransferase,
bone studies comprising proteins, albumin, calcium, phosphate and alkaline phosphatase, and
iron studies comprising iron, transferrin and ferritin.

1.9 Cascading

When the discretionary approach to the requesting and performance of clinical laboratory tests is adopted, particularly
where the clinician is encouraged to request small groups of
related tests, it is possible for the clinical laboratory to
perform additional relevant or required tests on the initiative
of the clinical chemistry laboratory staff.

This strategy, called cascading, is best illustrated by
reference to thyroid function tests. All patients on whom
thyroid function tests are requested might best be assessed by
measurement of the serum total thyroxine concentration. If
this was lower than the reference limit, serum thyrotrophin
assay would generally be carried out without a further request
and, if higher, serum triiodothyronine and an index of protein
binding such as free thyroxine index would be performed.

Such approaches cannot ever cover all possibilities (in the
example quoted above individuals on therapy or with triiodothyronine thyrotoxicosis would not be appropriately
investigated) and it is absolutely vital that, if the clinical
laboratory performs any cascading, very full clinical
information and drug therapy be provided with every request.

1.10 Clinical chemistry close to the patient

A recent trend is the performance of clinical laboratory tests on blood, serum or plasma close to the patient in wards, clinics or in surgeries of general practitioners. This important topic is dealt with in detail in Chapter 4.

Clinical chemistry tests of a very traditional nature, namely qualitative or semiquantitative urinalysis tests and similar tests such as that for faecal occult blood, have been and are still widely performed in situations close to the patient. The performance of such tests is not as easy as might be thought and the interpretation of the results is not always a simple matter. Recent publications document both laboratory and clinical aspects of this subject (*see* Further reading[2,10]) and the complementary text of Whitby, Percy-Robb and Smith mentioned in the preface does cover the subject in detail; it is therefore considered unnecessary to discuss these particular topics in depth in this text.

1.11 Emergency tests

One of the purposes of the clinical laboratory is to provide test results that are clinically useful *early* enough to influence decision making. Results of analytical procedures are reported at times after specimen receipt which are influenced by many factors including time of day, availability of equipment, the necessity to batch some tests to save money on expensive reagents, perceived clinical requirement and demands of individual clinicians. There is very little objective information on the turnaround times really required for optimal patient care. However, a small number of test results are required quickly in order to substantiate a diagnosis and/or to initiate treatment. These tests can be termed emergency, urgent or stat tests.

Clinical laboratories do adopt a wide variety of strategies to deal with such tests. Some require consultation at high level before performing a test. Separate laboratories or sections handling these particular tests may have been commissioned. Some have a widely publicized list of a small number of tests which are made freely available at all times. Outside normal working hours, staff may require to be called in to the clinical laboratory to perform such tests.

Whatever type of service is provided by the clinical laboratory, emergency tests should be requested only when really required for patient care because such services are expensive and the turnaround time of tests required in true emergency situations will be prolonged by submission of extra load to whatever system is in operation.

It should also be noted that laboratories may have to perform the analyses in less than ideal circumstances. The ideal is emergency and more usual tests being carried out on the same equipment using the same methodology and reagents in order to facilitate interpretation of all tests results produced. Emergency tests may be performed using different techniques and certain of these may have performance characteristics which are less than ideal.

1.12 Interpretation of numerical data

The process between the clinician initiating a request for clinical laboratory tests and then acting on the information received is complex. As illustrated in Fig. 1.1, there are many component steps and many individuals involved.

Errors of various types can occur at all stages of the process and, to interpret any numerical test results correctly, an appreciation of the real and potential sources of error and difficulty at each stage is required of all users and suppliers of clinical laboratory services.

In this chapter, the use of the clinical chemistry laboratory has been reviewed. In the rest of this text, in a logical order, the problems of preparation and documentation of the patient

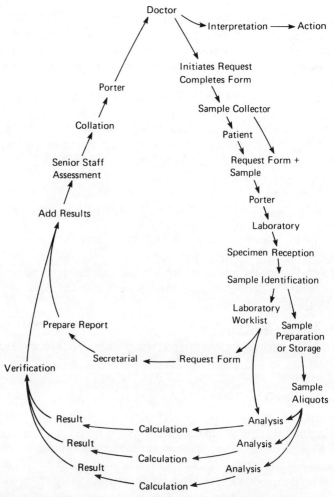

Fig. 1.1. The complex process between requesting a test and obtaining a result. From Fraser C.G. and Watkinson L.R. (1985) In Marks V. and Alberti K.G.M.M. Eds. *Clinical Biochemistry Nearer the Patient*, p.12. Churchill Livingstone, Edinburgh (with permission).

for specimen collection, the difficulties inherent in specimen collection, analytical considerations and the interpretation of numerical data in the light of knowledge of reference values, biological variability and the predictive value model will be discussed in detail.

1.13   Summary

The number of test results generated by clinical laboratories continues to increase each year. There are many logical reasons for this but there is no doubt that some tests are requested unnecessarily.

Test results are very useful in various aspects of diagnosis, management, screening, research, development and teaching. Consideration of the limitations of clinical laboratory tests in these situations would not only eliminate some of the large clinical laboratory workload but, more importantly, would lead to the more efficient and effective use of the clinical laboratory.

The process by which a test result is obtained is complex and an appreciation of the problems involved at each stage is a necessary prerequisite to the correct interpretation of clinical laboratory numerical test results.

Further reading

1 Connelly D.P. & Steele B. (1980) Laboratory utilization. Problems and solutions. *Archives of Pathology and Laboratory Medicine,* **104,** 59.
2 Fraser C.G. (1985) Urine analysis: current performance and strategies for improvement. *British Medical Journal,* **291,** 321.

3　Hardison J.E. (1979) To be complete. *New England Journal of Medicine,* **300,** 193.

4　Rang M. (1972) The Ulysses syndrome. *Journal of the Canadian Medical Association,* **106,** 122.

5　Speicher C.E. & Smith J.W. (1983) *Choosing Effective Laboratory Tests.* W.B. Saunders, Philadelphia.

6　Whitby L.G. (1968) Well – population screening. *British Journal of Hospital Medicine,* **2,** 79.

7　Whitehead T.P. & Wooton I.D.P. (1974) Biochemical profiles for hospital patients. *The Lancet,* **ii,** 1439.

8　Wilson J.M.G. & Junger G. (1968) *The Principles and Practice of Screening for Disease.* World Health Organization Public Health Papers No 34. WHO, Geneva.

9　Young D.S. (1979) Why is there a laboratory? In Young D.S. *et al.,* Eds. *Clinician and Chemist,* p. 3. American Association for Clinical Chemistry, Washington.

10　Zilva J.F. (1985) Is unselective biochemical urine testing cost effective? *British Medical Journal,* **291,** 323.

Chapter 2
Preanalytical factors

2.1 Introduction

Each laboratory result is obtained on a specimen from an *individual* patient and there are a great many factors which are unique to that patient which must be known and well documented before correct interpretation of results can be performed. The factors can be divided into four groups, namely (i) laboratory factors, (ii) endogenous factors (those that are outside the control of the individual such as age and sex), (iii) genetic factors and (iv) exogenous factors (those that are within, to a greater or lesser extent, the control of the individual). The first three groups of factors are discussed in detail in Chapter 5. The preanalytical exogenous factors, other than time factors which are considered in depth in Chapter 6, are the subject of this chapter.

The factors of importance are food and drink intake, alcohol intake, posture, stress, pregnancy, exercise, hospitalization, drug administration and previous medical and surgical care.

2.2 Food and drink intake

The effects of food and drink intake on clinical laboratory test results can be divided into at least three types, effects being found (i) after recent food or drink intake, (ii) on ingestion of particular foods or drinks that contain large amounts of a component to be assayed and (iii) due to long term dietary habits. This subject is discussed in detail by Young (*see* Further reading[6]).

Recent food intake

The findings documented in the literature on the effects of
meals or drinks on serum constituents are often conflicting
and, although statistically significant changes can be demonstrated for a number of analytes, it is unlikely that most of
these are of real significance in clinical contexts. This is well
documented by Statland and Winkel (*see* Further reading[3]).

However, certain changes are important. The lipaemia
which occurs after a meal can have significant effects on
clinical laboratory test results; these effects are very
dependent on laboratory methodology and the laboratory
should inform the clinician as to the validity or otherwise of
specimens with lipaemia. Possibly severe interpretative
problems can occur; for example, in assay of serum sodium
using traditional flame photometry, a 67-year-old male was
found to have a serum sodium of 124 mmol/l (reference
interval: 135–147 mmol/l). The specimen was very lipaemic
and the triglycerides present had lowered the water content of
the specimen. The sodium concentration in the aqueous
fraction of the plasma did lie within the reference interval, as
shown by analysis using direct ion selective electrode technology which gave a result of 137 mmol/l. A similar finding
occurs when very high concentrations of protein (> 120 g/l)
are present, the aqueous component of the plasma being
reduced. Laboratories can overcome the problems of
lipaemia by either ultracentrifugation or by enzymatic
cleavage of triglycerides prior to analysis.

The changes in plasma glucose levels which follow meals are
widely appreciated. Ingestion of caffeine, in tea, coffee and
many carbonated beverages has striking effects on certain
constituents, plasma cortisol rising to 140–159% of the basal
level after 3 hours and urinary catecholamines being significantly increased.

These potential problems could be avoided by specimen

collection in a standardized manner when the patient is in the fasting state; this is obviously not always possible in real clinical practice. Moreover, fasting, particularly if prolonged, has some interesting effects on clinical laboratory tests, including an increase in serum bilirubins concentration (on average 240% after 48 hours) and, in some women, a fall in plasma glucose to less than 2.2 mmol/l without concomitant symptoms of hypoglycaemia.

Ingestion of particular foods and drinks

A number of foods may cause specific analytical problems. Urinary 5-hydroxyindoleacetic acid excretion, for example, is significantly increased by ingestion of serotonin containing fruits such as bananas. Urinary hydroxymethoxymandelic acid excretion may be elevated by a diet rich in vanillin containing materials. Certain tests for faecal blood will give positive results when a meat-rich diet is consumed. When such effects are known, dietary restrictions should be imposed prior to specimen collection.

Long term habits

There is considerable evidence that the type of food ingested has marked effects on clinical laboratory test results. The excretion of a large number of urinary constituents, for example, sodium, chloride, potassium and phosphate, is dependent upon intake in addition to the state of nutrition. Adoption of a diet rich in protein leads to higher levels of serum urea, cholesterol and phosphate. In nutritionally deprived individuals, the total serum proteins and albumin are reduced as are cholesterol and triglycerides concentrations and the activities of certain serum enzymes, notably alkaline phosphatase. These factors undoubtedly contribute a great deal to the differences in reference values quoted for different groups in different parts of the world (*see* Chapter 5).

2.3 Alcohol intake

Alcohol intake causes a number of changes in clinical laboratory test results. However, the situation is complex and the changes are dependent on the type of individual (abuser or nonabuser of alcohol), the time of specimen collection after intake of the alcohol, the quantity of alcohol consumed and the biological response of the individual. Many studies have been performed assessing the test results found in abusers of alcohol in order to attempt to delineate clinical laboratory tests useful for the evaluation of abuse. These studies are complicated by the factors listed above, the difficulties of estimating alcohol intake and intrinsic intraindividual biological variation (*see* Chapter 6). Certain serum enzyme activities are, however, elevated even after a single ethanol challenge particularly alkaline phosphatase, creatine kinase, aspartate aminotransferase and lactate dehydrogenase. Serum gamma-glutamyltransferase activity is also elevated in this situation as well as in the majority of alcohol abusers. In addition, elevated concentrations of serum urate and HDL-cholesterol are found in such individuals. Different effects may be seen in abusers and nonabusers, for example, intake of alcohol in the abuser may occasionally cause marked hypoglycaemia (with concurrent lactic acidosis) whereas, in the nonabuser, large quantities of alcohol lead to increased plasma glucose levels.

2.4   Posture

When an individual changes from a lying to a standing position, body water shifts from the vascular compartment to the interstitial compartment. This shift in body water leads to marked changes in the components of plasma which cannot shift compartments, that is, large molecules, small molecules bound to large molecules and cells. Thus, plasma or serum levels of the following rise by 8 to 10% when an individual stands up: proteins; albumin; cholesterol; bilirubins; triglycerides; aspartate and alanine aminotransferases; alkaline and acid phosphatase; other enzymes; iron; hormones bound to carrier proteins.

Serum calcium levels rise by 4–5% in this situation because only about 50% of the total calcium is bound to plasma albumin. Similarly, serum or plasma drug levels change on adoption of a different posture, the magnitude of the change being related to the fraction of drug bound to carrier proteins.

A change in posture also has significant effects on the levels of plasma hormones associated with control of blood volume and pressure, for example, plasma renin activity and aldosterone are doubled in the ambulant compared with the resting individual.

If a patient is sitting for specimen collection, the changes seen in the results of clinical laboratory tests affected by posture will be 60–70% of the effects described here that occur upon adoption of a standing position.

There is no doubt that the effects of postural changes on clinical laboratory test results do cause some problems in interpretation, particularly in the assessment of serial results obtained on specimens from an individual patient who has been, for example, an inpatient and an outpatient. Some clinical laboratories quote different reference values for inpatients and outpatients but those adopting this strategy often quote appropriate values for a few constituents such as serum proteins, albumin and calcium; others are also affected.

2.5 Stress

There are many causes of stress seen in hospital patients and others who seek medical advice. These include mental stress from fear or anxiety and physical stress from pain or surgical trauma. The responses seen in clinical laboratory test results are similar, irrespective of the source of the stress. The hormonal response to stress causes increases in the following: plasma cortisol; urinary oxogenic steroids; plasma growth hormone; plasma prolactin; serum cholesterol; urinary catecholamines.

It is important to recognize that even the anxiety and pain experienced by certain individuals on being subjected to venepuncture can elicit this response. This is particularly relevant to assessment of plasma cortisol levels because rises up to ten-fold can be seen. An example of the response in plasma cortisol levels seen in repeated venepuncture of a patient compared to the levels found when multiple specimens were taken via a venous catheter are shown in Fig. 2.1. Partly as a result of this phenomenon, suspected diseases of the hypothalamic-pituitary-adrenal axis are best investigated by dynamic function tests.

Stress has effects on other analytes. For example, the stress of myocardial infarction or major surgery leads to a fall in the serum iron which becomes significant after 24 hours, a fall in transferrin after 32–40 hours and a rise in ferritin after 40–48 hours. This has ramifications, not only for interpretation of test results, but also for specimen collection in that, if it is wished to use clinical chemistry test results to aid in the assessment of iron status, specimens must be collected within 24 hours after the myocardial infarction has taken place or

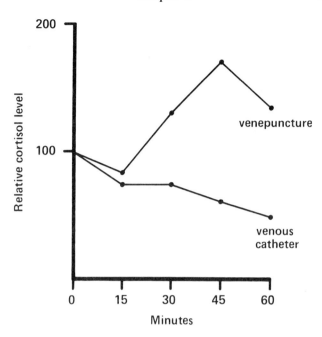

Fig. 2.1. Plasma cortisol levels in a patient; specimens taken by stressful venepuncture and via an indwelling catheter. Modified from James V.H.T. and Landon J. *Hypothalamic–Pituitary–Adrenal Function Tests.* CIBA Laboratories, Horsham.

before surgery has been undertaken. It has recently also been shown that, contrary to existing dogma which states that specimens for lipids analyses cannot be collected after stressful events such as myocardial infarction, serum triglycerides levels do not change significantly after this stress. Levels of serum cholesterol, low density lipoproteins and high density lipoproteins, although they do fall significantly, are not in fact significantly different on day one, day two or three months after infarction. Thus, the lipid state can be assessed satisfactorily during the first 48 hours after infarction but no later.

As a general rule, when a test result is not truly requested for immediate diagnosis or treatment, the specimens should not be collected when the patient has been stressed by disease or surgical intervention because of the many effects of stress on clinical laboratory test results.

2.6 Pregnancy

Pregnancy is discussed in this particular chapter because, unlike age, sex and body mass (*see* Chapter 5), the changes in clinical laboratory test results seen in this particular physiological state are only temporary. The many biological responses to pregnancy have been described in detail by Lind (*see* Further reading[2]). These may be considered as two groups, the nonhormonal and the hormonal.

During pregnancy, the plasma volume rises but not in a linear fashion; there is little rise during the first 10 weeks of pregnancy and then a rise to a maximum of an increase of approximately 30% at about 30 weeks. The erythrocyte volume also increases but in a slightly different pattern and to a lesser extent. These changes are not related. The overall effect is sometimes considered to be a *dilution* effect, as seen in the serum urea, creatinine, proteins and albumin from a typical 30 week pregnant woman, shown in Table 2.1.

This dilution explanation is not correct because, although the levels of some constituents, such as proteins, albumin, urea, creatinine, iron, sodium, potassium, calcium and magnesium do fall significantly and the falls of the first five listed are of an order of 10–20%, the levels of certain commonly assayed serum constituents such as phosphate, aspartate aminotransferase and alanine aminotransferase do not show any significant changes.

Table 2.1.

Constituent	Result	Usual adult reference interval
Sodium	139 mmol/l	135–147
Potassium	4.0 mmol/l	3.5–5.0
Chloride	107 mmol/l	95–105
Bicarbonate	23 mmol/l	21–28
Urea	3.9 mmol/l	3.3–6.6
Creatinine	52 μmol/l	44–150
Calcium	2.25 mmol/l	2.15–2.65
Phosphate	1.21 mmol/l	0.8–1.55
Proteins	50 g/l	65–80
Albumin	27 g/l	36–50

Moreover, many serum constituents rise during pregnancy including caeruloplasmin (by 100%), transferrin (by 25%), other proteins of the $alpha_1$, $alpha_2$ and beta-globulin classes including the lipoproteins, which is reflected in rises in the serum cholesterol and triglycerides levels, and in certain enzymes, notably those produced in the placenta such as alkaline phosphatase. Certain of these changes are shown in Fig. 2.2.

Thus the changes seen in pregnancy in nonhormonal constituents are many and varied and are not due simply to dilutional effects but are an integral component of this complex biological event. As a consequence, reference values appropriate to the pregnant women require to be used as interpretative aids and, in many cases, the values must be stratified according to the stage of gestation.

Many hormonal changes are seen in the plasma and urine during pregnancy; indeed, assay of a number of these provide diagnostic information. Particularly important to recognize are those shown in Fig. 2.3. For clinical purposes, monitoring of serial results in an individual patient and assessment of changes is more often important and more valuable than performance of a single assay and comparison of the test result with reference values, even if correctly stratified. Serum levels of other hormones in pregnancy must be interpreted carefully; the higher levels of serum thyroxine and cortisol for

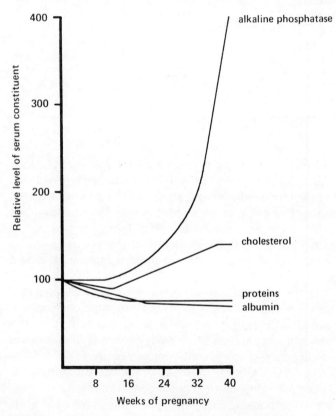

Fig. 2.2. Changes seen in some serum constituents during pregnancy.

example are mainly due to the higher levels of hormone binding proteins seen in pregnancy.

2.7   Exercise

Physical exercise has many effects on clinical laboratory test results and these have been reviewed in detail by Statland and

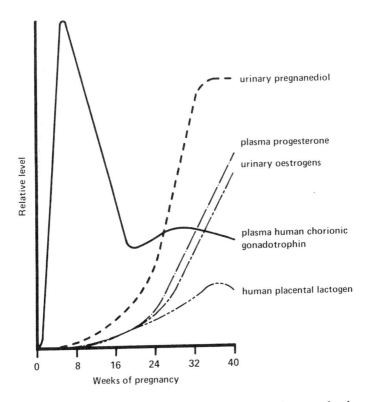

Fig. 2.3.   Changes seen in some plasma and urinary hormone levels during pregnancy.

Winkel (*see* Further reading[4]). The effects depend on a number of factors including the type and amount of exercise undertaken and whether the individual is trained or not.

After exercise, serum activities of enzymes present in muscle cells, notably creatine kinase, lactate dehydrogenase and aspartate aminotransferase, are increased and data obtained in four healthy young men after one hour of exercise are shown in Fig. 2.4. The increases seen peak some hours after exercise and are still evident after more than one day.

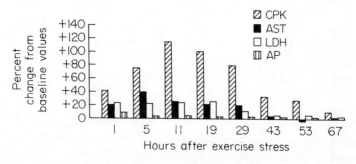

Fig. 2.4. The mean percent change for each of four enzyme activity values in four healthy young men after 1 hour of moderate to strenuous exercise. From King S., Statland B.E. and Savory J. (1970) *Clinica chimica acta,* **72,** 211 (with permission).

Certain hormone levels increase after exercise, notably growth hormone, this fact being utilized in the exercise stress test for the investigation of growth hormone deficiency in children, cortisol, prolactin, plasma renin activity and catecholamines. Moreover, prolonged physical training does have marked effects; in young men, plasma levels of testosterone, androstenedione and luteotrophin increased by about 25% after six months of effort.

A number of other constituents whose analyses are often requested by clinicians are affected by exercise including serum urea, creatinine, urate, calcium and magnesium. These changes, although statistically significant, are not thought likely to cause marked problems in interpretation of clinical laboratory test results.

2.8 Hospitalization

Hospital clinicians and clinical laboratory staff are generally dealing with hospitalized patients. It should be remembered that diet, posture, stress and activity have the effects on clinical laboratory test results described earlier. All of these preanalytical factors are likely to be modified on hospitalization. In addition, hospitalized patients are prone to show some characteristic general responses to illness including lower serum iron and total thyroxine and elevated serum triglycerides.

Immobilization itself has some interesting biological effects including increased calcium and phosphate excretion but no effects on the serum levels of these are seen unless there is increased bone turnover such as occurs in Paget's disease or in patients with fractures.

2.9 Drug administration

Drugs have many effects on clinical laboratory tests results and the magnitude of this problem is evidenced by the fact that it has recently been suggested that there are over 25000 references in the published literature that document the effects of drugs and other factors which cause interpretative problems. It is therefore impossible to describe all the potential sources of difficulties here. It is important to realize, however, that there are very complete lists of such effects in both written and computerized format (*see* Further reading[5,7]). The clinical chemist usually has access to such literature sources and it is good practice for these staff to be consulted either before a test result considered to be inappropriate has been reported or after the clinician has considered a result to be worthy of suspicion and subsequently notified the clinical laboratory.

The effects of drugs are of two different types. Drugs or their metabolites may interfere with the analytical method used by the laboratory; these *in vitro* effects are often very dependent on the precise methodology used in the individual laboratory. Drugs may also lead to physiological effects which cause changes in clinical laboratory test results; these *in vivo* effects are the most commonly encountered drug-test interactions accounting for about 80%.

Some examples of commonly encountered *in vitro* effects follow in order to show the spectrum seen in practice.

Paracetamol causes increased plasma glucose levels of approximately 1.4 mmol/l per mmol/l paracetamol when the assay is performed on a Yellow Springs glucose analyser; no such interference is seen with other analytical systems. Certain cephalosporin antibiotics cause elevated serum creatinine levels when colorimetric reactions using alkaline picrate are used; not all antibiotics of this type react in this manner and the degree of interference is very dependent on the exact chemical conditions of the reaction. A high intake and consequent output of vitamin C can cause many drug-test interactions including the finding of false negative results for urinary glucose and blood with reagent dip-sticks. Assays of 5-hydroxyindoleacetic acid using the nitrosonaphthol technique are elevated by naproxin and paracetamol but lowered by phenothiazines. A metabolite of propanolol, namely 4-hydroxypropanolol, causes positive interference in urinary hydroxymethoxymandelic acid assays. Labetalol hydrochloride leads to falsely elevated urinary metanephrine results. Administration of dextran intravenously as a plasma expander causes falsely elevated results for plasma proteins in assays using the Biuret technique and nutrient solutions such as Intralipid® and Liposyn® given intravenously in critically ill patients cause several analytical problems with certain laboratory techniques. Prednisolone cross reacts with most antisera currently used in immunoassays for plasma cortisol and administration leads to artificially high serum levels.

The more important *in vivo* group of drug-test interactions may be classified in a number of ways; only the most common effects will be described here based upon the class of drug.

Oral contraceptives have many effects on the results of critical laboratory tests; these are dependent on the type of pill, particularly on the biological activity and on whether oestrogen or progestogen or both are present. Oestrogens can cause some degree of impairment of glucose tolerance and elevate serum triglycerides possibly due to induction of hepatic microsomal enzymes. Oestrogens also cause many changes in plasma proteins including lower levels of albumin and haptoglobin and increases in many proteins particularly transport proteins including thyroxine binding globulin, transcortin, sex hormone binding globulin, transferrin and other proteins including caeruloplasmin and certain of the proteins involved in the blood coagulation process. As a result of the increases in the transport proteins caused by oestrogen stimulation of hepatic synthesis, many clinical laboratory test results such as plasma cortisol, total thyroxine and triiodothyronine will be high; the free hormone levels will be within the reference intervals. In some women, oral contraceptives may cause changes in the test results obtained to aid in the assessment of liver function. Aspartate and alanine aminotransferase activities in serum may be transiently raised, serum alkaline phosphatase and gamma-glutamyltransferase activities may be somewhat increased and occasionally a clinically evident jaundice with elevated serum and urinary bilirubin and appropriate changes in enzyme activities may occur.

Thiazide diuretics, in addition to furosemide and aceta-zolamide, often cause hyperuricaemia. Thiazides can have other effects including causing hypercalcaemia.

Narcotic drugs including morphine and codeine cause hyperamylasaemia, hyperamylasuria and hyperlipasaemia because of their effect on the sphincter of Oddi and may cause transient increases in the serum activities of enzymes present in the hepatocytes.

Phenytoin, barbiturates and most other antiepileptic drugs, through induction of hepatic microsomal enzymes, cause marked increases in serum gamma-glutamyltransferase activity.

It is vital that these *in vivo* drug-test interactions be recognized because failure to do so leads to patients often being misclassified as diseased, treated when this is unnecessary or subjected to further clinical laboratory and other investigations which are not required.

2.10 Previous medical and surgical care

In addition to prescribed drugs causing problems in the interpretation of clinical laboratory test results, medical or surgical care can cause similar difficulties. The significant general effects of stress and hospitalization which have been described earlier in this chapter must be remembered.

The classic example quoted in many textbooks is that palpation of the prostate leads to an increase in the serum acid phosphatase activity. Recent data suggest that this is in reality a myth that has been perpetrated over the years without systematic study and only occurs rarely. In contrast, prostatectomy does cause increased serum activities and this test should not be requested for seven days after operation.

Intramuscular injections can cause problems in the interpretation of the results of assays of serum enzyme activities.

Serum creatine kinase, lactate dehydrogenase, aldolase and aspartate aminotransferase activities are all elevated after such procedures. Surgery can have similar consequences.

After blood transfusion, serum bilirubins levels may be elevated transiently presumably from the extra load presented to the liver. Moreover, specimens of blood taken after transfusion reflect, on analysis, the composition of the mixture of that present and that given rather than the true homeostatic state of the patient.

2.11 Other factors

Many specimens submitted to the clinical laboratory for analysis are taken from patients who have diseases which cause levels of analytes in body fluids to be different from the apparently healthy. Such analytes may cause difficulties in interpretation of test results. Examples include high levels of triglycerides which cause lipaemia and high levels of proteins which can lead to factitious hyponatraemia as discussed earlier. Bilirubins present in sera from jaundiced patients can cause interference in a number of clinical laboratory test procedures such as the falsely low results for plasma calcium found using semiautomated fluorimetric techniques; the effects of icterus are very method dependent and good liaison between clinician and laboratory is again essential for correct interpretation of results and avoidance of unnecessary treatment or further laboratory tests. Acetoacetate present in the plasma of patients with diabetic ketoacidosis can cause markedly elevated apparent levels of serum creatinine with a number of colorimetric methods based upon the commonly used techniques. A large intake of alcohol will, as for methanol, isopropanol and propylene glycol, lead to accumulation of osmotically active particles in the plasma and, as a result, the measured plasma osmolality will be very much higher than the calculated osmolarity which is often simply assessed as $2\times[Na^+]+2\times[K^+]+[urea]+[glucose]$ in mmol/l. An unusually low anion gap, calculated as $([Na^+]+[K^+])-([Cl^-]+[HCO_3^-])$, is occasionally found when paraprotein, assumed to have negative charge, is present.

Other factors may be important to recognize. One significant example is that patients may not have a body temperature of 37°C. However, modern equipment for the analysis of blood pH and partial pressures of gases the measurements at 37°C. If the patient is hypothermic, the pH will be higher than the Pco_2 and Po_2 lower. The opposite effects will be seen in patients with fever.

Although not universally accepted, many would correct the found results by application of the following formulae:

> pH: −0.02 per °C rise
> Pco_2: +0.7 kPa (5 mmHg) per °C rise
> Po_2: +0.5 kPa (4 mmHg) per °C rise

Some case studies showing these effects have been documented by Fraser and Watkinson (*see* Further reading[1]).

Many other less important preanalytical factors affect the results of laboratory tests and the detailed article by Young (*see* Further reading[7]) is highly recommended as an information source should problems be thought to exist.

2.12 Summary

Each patient on whom clinical laboratory tests are performed is unique and much must be known about the individual and the lifestyle adopted by the individual before laboratory test results can be interpreted correctly. The factors of which it is important to gain knowledge include the previous food and drink intake, both recent and habitual, whether any particular food or drink taken will cause difficulties with the specific tests to be performed, alcohol intake, the posture at the time of specimen collection, stress, whether the patient is pregnant, whether exercise is regularly taken or has recently been engaged in, the effects of hospitalization, the drugs that have been taken, the effects of previous medical and surgical care and other factors.

Further reading

1   Fraser C.G. & Watkinson L.R. (1985) Patient, specimen and analysis as potential sources of error. *In* Marks V. & Alberti K.G.M.M. Eds. *Clinical Biochemistry Near the Patient,* pp. 11–33. Churchill Livingstone, Edinburgh.

2   Lind T. (1980) Clinical chemistry of pregnancy. *Advances in Clinical Chemistry,* **21,** 1.

3   Statland B.E. & Winkel P. (1977) Effects of preanalytical factors on the intraindividual variation of analytes in the blood of healthy individuals: consideration of preparation of the subject and time of venepuncture. *CRC Critical Reviews in Clinical Laboratory Sciences,* **8,** 105.

4   Statland B.E. & Winkel P. (1981) Response of clinical chemistry quantity values to selected physical, dietary, and smoking activities. *Progress in Clinical Pathology,* **8,** 25.

5   Tryding N. *et al.* Eds. (1983) *Drug Effects in Clinical Chemistry,* 3rd ed. Apoteksbolaget, Stockholm.

6   Young D.S. (1979) Biological variability. In Brown S.S., Mitchell F.L. & Young D.S. Eds. *Chemical Diagnosis of Disease,* pp. 1–113. Elsevier, Amsterdam.

7   Young D.S., Pestaner L. & Gibberman V. (1975) Effects of drugs on clinical laboratory tests. *Clinical Chemistry,* **21,** ID.

Chapter 3

Specimen Collection

3.1. Introduction

In order to obtain clinical laboratory test results which do not pose significant problems in interpretation, specimens must be collected from a *correctly prepared* patient and with full knowledge of those *circumstances prevailing at the time of specimen collection* which may be relevant (Chapter 2). Furthermore, the *time* at which specimens should be collected to facilitate interpretation must be carefully considered (Chapter 6). Collection of specimens is also not without difficulties and the correct techniques for collection, transport and storage, and the problems that can arise are the subjects of this chapter.

3.2. Patient identification

Although it appears self-evident, it is essential to ensure that all specimens and request forms are clearly marked with unambiguous patient identification and that the specimen is indeed being collected from the correct patient, particularly when the patient is unable for any reason to communicate and verbal assurance of identity cannot be gained.

Mistakes do occur, often when two patients with similar names are geographically close. As one example, Thomas W and James W were both patients in the same ward. Test results were obtained on serum specimens as shown in Table 3.1. It was obvious to the clinical chemist responsible for verification of results that an error had been made and, on attempting to find the source of the problem, it appeared highly likely that

Table 3.1.

		Thomas		James	
Constituent	*Units*	*Day 1*	*Day 2*	*Day 1*	*Day 2*
Sodium	mmol/l	140	134	134	140
Potassium	mmol/l	4.6	4.6	4.4	3.8
Chloride	mmol/l	110	96	96	109
Bicarbonate	mmol/l	21	30	31	22
Urea	mmol/l	15.5	6.8	5.6	15.7
Calcium	mmol/l	2.25	2.06	2.22	2.07
Albumin	g/l	35	26	28	32
Phospate	mmol/l	1.38	1.24	1.27	1.20
Alkaline phosphatase	mmol/l	109	376	431	100
Bilirubins	mmol/l	12	16	20	10
Proteins	g/l	59	49	54	51
Creatinine	μmol/l	250	62	65	242

the specimens were simply taken from the wrong patients. Similar errors can occur at a number of stages in the process of obtaining a result, for example, through transcription mistakes or by incorrect placing of specimens on an instrument sampling rack.

Errors can also arise where timed urine collections are being performed simultaneously on a number of patients in the same ward. It is all too easy for a specimen passed by one patient to be added to the collection of another patient, especially when the specimens are all kept together in a refrigerator or side room.

3.3 Blood collection

The techniques of specimen collection will not be detailed in this text. These are best acquired through experience once taught by a skilled individual and, if a description is sought, the techniques are excellently described in the book by Slockblower and Blumenfeld (*see* Further reading[5]). In this section, the many potential difficulties inherent in blood collection will be described.

Blood collection site

Most specimens submitted to the clinical laboratory for analysis are venous blood specimens collected by conventional venepuncture using either traditional syringes and needles, with subsequent transfer of blood to an appropriate container, or using evacuated tube systems, the tubes containing any anticoagulant or preservative required.

The venous blood specimen must be collected from an appropriate site. Many hospitalized patients are being given intravenous therapy. Blood specimens should not normally be taken from sites proximal to the infusion on the same limb otherwise the specimen collected is a mixture of blood and the intravenous solution given. For example, a specimen collected in such a manner from a patient being given dextrose (glucose) showed results shown in Table 3.2.

Table 3.2.

Constituent	Units	Result	Reference interval
Sodium	mmol/l	106	135–147
Potassium	mmol/l	3.1	3.5–5.0
Chloride	mmol/l	92	95–105
Bicarbonate	mmol/l	16	21–28
Urea	mmol/l	3.0	3.3–6.6
Creatinine	μmol/l	80	44–150
Calcium	mmol/l	1.48	2.15–2.65
Phosphate	mmol/l	0.58	0.80–1.55

The dilutional effect of the dextrose solution is obvious. When isotonic saline is given, the effect may not be quite so obvious but the chloride level is usually very markedly elevated and other constituents low, often in the presence of eunatraemia. In a patient known to have previously had chronic obstructive airways disease, serum bicarbonate of 36 mmol/l, chloride of 86 mmol/l, potassium of 2.6 mmol/l, urea of 11.0 mmol/l and creatinine of 135 μmol/l, the results shown in Table 3.3 were seen, demonstrating this type of error.

Table 3.3.

Constituent	Units	Result	Reference interval
Sodium	mmol/l	146	135–147
Potassium	mmol/l	1.6	3.5–5.0
Chloride	mmol/l	124	95–105
Bicarbonate	mmol/l	15	21–28
Urea	mmol/l	4.5	3.3–6.6
Creatinine	μmol/l	50	44–150
Calcium	mmol/l	1.16	2.15–2.65
Phosphate	mmol/l	0.24	0.80–1.55

This phenomenon is also seen when patients are undergoing dialysis and specimens are erroneously collected from the venous side of the dialyser.

Contamination

The preparation of the specimen collection site is important. Capillary plasma glucose levels apparently can be elevated by prior handling of confectionary. Swabbing with alcohol prior to venepuncture can cause elevated blood alcohol levels if ethanol is a component of the swab fluid and low results if isopropanol, the usual analytical internal standard, is used.

Perhaps the most relevant example of specimen contamination is the effect of air bubbles and froth on pH and blood gas
analyses. The size of bubble is of little importance and Po_2
levels rise after three minutes if air is present and glass
syringes are used.

Anticoagulation

A further error often made when blood specimens are collected is the inappropriate use of anticoagulants or preservatives. Commonly used in clinical chemistry are: lithium
heparin (12 units/ml blood); K₂EDTA (2.0 mg/ml blood);
fluoride/oxalate (1.0 mg sodium fluoride plus 3.0 mg potassium oxalate/ml blood).

The use of lithium heparin as anticoagulant has advantages
over the use of serum in that (i) the time taken for clot
formation and retraction and (ii) the difficulties of poor clot
formation in some plastic containers are avoided. However, it
must be realized that certain analyses such as protein
electrophoresis and some immunoassays cannot be performed
on plasma, plasma gives a less optically clear specimen for
analysis and lithium assays cannot be carried out on heparinized plasma unless the sodium salt is used. Although it is often
assumed that heparinized plasma and serum are interchange-
able, there are statistically significant differences between the
results obtained on these two types of specimen for many
common tests. The differences are generally small but should
be borne in mine as a contributory source of variation when
specimens of both types are taken from the individual patient.
The specimen type generally used by the clinical laboratory
will also affect the reference values quoted (*see* Chapter 5).
Reference values for plasma will be somewhat lower than for
serum for those constituents present at high levels in
erythrocytes, notably potassium, phosphate, aspartate

aminotransferase and lactate dehydrogenase, because the clotting process presumably causes some release of these constituents into the serum. Heparin is used when arterial blood is collected for pH and blood gas analyses and prepacked syringes containing liquid heparin are available for this purpose. Irrespective of the variability between brands and between different batches of the same brand, if all excess heparin is not expelled from the syringe before specimen collection, decreased pH and increased P_{CO_2} are found; the effect on P_{O_2} is variable. Use of heparin lyophilized in the collection syringe eliminates this problem.

Blood collected into K_2EDTA tubes cannot be used for certain analyses. Although it is usual for clinical laboratory staff to reject specimens in inappropriate containers, sometimes ward-based staff inadvertently tip some specimen collected in such a container into what appears to be the correct container. For example, a serum specimen analysed gave the following results shown in Table 3.4

The results were viewed with suspicion by the clinical

Table 3.4.

Constituent	Units	Result	Reference interval
Sodium	mmol/l	140	135–147
Potassium	mmol/l	6.8	3.5–5.0
Chloride	mmol/l	101	95–105
Bicarbonate	mmol/l	24	21–28
Urea	mmol/l	5.1	3.3–6.6
Creatinine	μmol/l	87	44–150
Calcium	mmol/l	1.67	2.15–2.65
Phosphate	mmol/l	1.31	0.80–1.55
Proteins	g/l	70	65–80
Albumin	g/l	49	36–50
Alkaline phosphatase	U/l	58	25–120

chemist who initiated collection of a further specimen. On analysis all results fell within the reference intervals and the alkaline phosphatase activity was 86 U/l. K_2EDTA, in addition to elevating the potassium, chelates calcium causing factitious hypocalcaemia and also chelates magnesium, a necessary co-factor for alkaline phosphatase.

Fluoride/oxalate contamination causes similar errors, including elevation of sodium and potassium and lowering of calcium.

Other more subtle effects can be seen. Many of these are dependent on the exact methodology used by the laboratory.

It should be remembered that specimens for submission to more than one clinical laboratory may be collected at the same time and unusual inappropriate anticoagulant effects seen. For example, analysis of a serum specimen gave the following results shown in Table 3.5.

Table 3.5.

Constituent	Units	Result	Reference interval
Sodium	mmol/l	175	135–147
Potassium	mmol/l	3.4	3.5–5.0
Chloride	mmol/l	86	95–105
Bicarbonate	mmol/l	18	21–28
Urea	mmol/l	7.4	3.3–6.6
Creatinine	μmol/l	77	44–150
Calcium	mmol/l	1.97	2.15–2.65
Phosphate	mmol/l	0.82	0.80–1.55
Proteins	g/l	55	65–80
Albumin	g/l	30	36–50

The obviously inappropriate serum sodium result was eventually traced to contamination by sodium citrate which was used by the haematology laboratory as an anticoagulant for specimens for clotting studies.

When evacuated tubes are used for multiple specimen collection, contamination of one specimen from the anticoagulant of the previous specimen tube can occur. It is therefore important to consider carefully the order in which specimens are collected using this technique and serum collected before tubes containing additives. When additives are required, the recommended order of specimen collection is into tubes containing citrate, heparin, K_2EDTA and oxalate/ fluoride (*see* Further reading[1]).

Special requirements

For certain analyses performed by the clinical laboratory, very special collection conditions are required. For example, for specimens for adrenocorticotrophin and plasma renin activity assays are usually collected into cooled containers containing the appropriate preservative.

Haemolysis

Incorrect technique, including traumatic venepuncture, use of dirty or wet tubes and forcing blood through the needle, can lead to haemolysis. The average compositions of plasma and erythrocytes have marked differences, shown in Table 3.6.

When haemolysis is present, incorrect elevated levels of potassium, phosphate, lactate dehydrogenase and aspartate aminotransferase will be found. Moreover, the haemoglobin present can, by virtue of its intrinsic colour, interfere in many colorimetric assays used in the clinical laboratory; the degree of interference is very method dependent.

Table 3.6.

Constituent	Units	Plasma	Erythrocytes
Sodium	mmol/l	140	16
Potassium	mmol/l	4	100
Chloride	mmol/l	104	52
Bicarbonate	mmol/l	25	10
Urea	mmol/l	5.5	4.0
Calcium	mmol/l	2.50	0.25
Phosphate	mmol/l	1.2	4.2
Glucose	mmol/l	5.0	4.1
Cholesterol	mmol/l	6.0	4.3
Lactate dehydrogenase	U/l	180	30 000
Aspartate aminotransferase	U/l	25	500

Tourniquet application

The application of a tourniquet to aid specimen collection causes venous occlusion. The resulting raised intravenous pressure causes water, small ions and molecules to move into the extravascular space and large molecules and cells are retained intravenously. The levels of all proteins, including serum enzymes, and protein-bound moeities including calcium, bilirubin, cholesterol, triglycerides, thyroxine, cortisol, other hormones and drugs, can be raised to high or equivocal levels in a short time (*see* Further reading[6]). Some examples are shown in Fig. 3.1. It has also been suggested that prolonged stasis can lead to local hypoxia which results in leakage of erythrocyte contents and a picture similar to haemolysis may be seen.

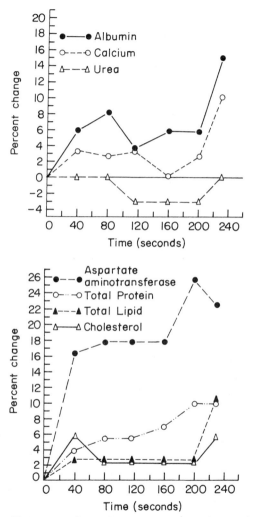

Fig. 3.1. Percentage change in some serum constituents during continuous tourniquet application. From Statland B.E. *et al.* (1974) *Clinical Chemistry*, **20**, 1518 (with permission).

Capillary blood collection

The small blood volume of young children and neonates, particularly those which are premature, mean that in addition to special care being taken with all aspects of specimen collection and handling, heel puncture is the generally performed procedure. In addition, capillary specimen collection from the distal phalanges of the fingers is often performed in older children and in adults when only small specimens are required or venepuncture proves difficult. Serum or plasma obtained from capillary blood does have some differences compared to those from venous blood. Glucose levels are higher and potassium, proteins and calcium lower by amounts that could be clinically significant. Moreover, capillary specimens have generally a higher level of haemolysis with the resulting problems detailed earlier in this chapter.

Timing

For many constituents analysed in the clinical laboratory, the time of specimen collection is crucial as is discussed in Chapter 6. A further consideration, not detailed there, is that, as a general rule, specimens for assay of therapeutic drugs should be taken before a patient receives medication rather than afterwards. This is not always practical, but specimens should never be taken within seven hours following medication with digoxin, lithium and valproate. It is also important to note that, after changes in therapeutic regime, adequate time should be allowed for the new steady state to be established (theophylline: 2 days; valproate: 4 days; lithium: 5 days; others: 1–3 weeks). Specimens taken before the establishment of equilibrium conditions may give information which is difficult to interpret correctly.

3.4   Urine collection

Urine may be collected as a random specimen, an early morning specimen or as a timed collection. The first two types are generally used for urinalysis and for a few assays performed in the clinical chemistry laboratory, notably electrolytes and osmolality. The many problems inherent in the apparently simple technique of urinalysis have been recently reviewed in detail (*see* Further reading[3]). Clinical chemistry laboratories more often require the collection of timed specimens.

The most crucial two points regarding collection of timed specimens are that (i) the patient must be given clear unambiguous instructions as to how to collect the specimen and (ii) the correct preservative and/or stabilizer must be present.

Simple instructions of the following form should suffice for the collection of the traditional 24 hour collection and these can easily be modified for other types of collection:

Use the bottle provided.

At the start of the 24 hour collection empty the bladder and DISCARD THIS SPECIMEN OF URINE. Note the exact time on the bottle label.

Collect all the urine passed during the next 24 hours and put it into a bottle which should be kept in a cool place or preferably in a refrigerator at 4°C.

On the following day, at EXACTLY the time noted on the label on the previous day, empty the bladder and add this urine to the collection bottle. Note the EXACT time on the bottle label.

If any urine is discarded in error, a new collection should be started.

If a bowel movement is anticipated during the collection period, collect the urine first and add it to the collection bottle. If the urine is contaminated, a new collection should be started.

Urine collections may require preservation in order to prevent bacterial growth. In addition, stabilization may be required to ensure that the constituents to be analysed do not degrade. Ideally, one agent could be used for all specimens but this ideal cannot be fulfilled. There is not a great deal of published work objectively evaluating preservatives and stabilizers and it is highly likely that many of the statements made in text books and many of the practices currently adopted by laboratories are not based upon real scientific evidence but are traditional. For example, glacial acetic acid is often recommended as the ideal preservative for urinary 5-hydroxyindoleacetic acid; however, in nitrosonapthol methods with extraction, this preservative causes marked negative interference.

A detailed study of preservatives and stabilizers has recently been performed by Shephard and Mazzachi in Australia (*see* Further reading[4]) and the recommendations are shown in Table 3.7.

Incorrect stabilization can cause severe problems in interpretation of results. For example, calcium, phosphate and oxalate may precipitate out of solution if the urine is not acidic and urate may precipitate out of solution if the urine is not alkaline; erroneously low results would be found. These situations can be retrieved in the clinical chemistry laboratory because, if the urine is well mixed and the pH adjusted appropriately, the precipitated material will redissolve. In contrast, hydroxymethoxymandelic acid and 5-hydroxyindoleacetic acid must be collected into acid because they degrade on standing at appropriate pH. However, it must be recognized that the appropriate amount of stabilizer must be present since an excess could alter the pH so much that the analytical technique could be affected.

3.5   Cerebrospinal fluid collection

Cerebrospinal fluid, normally collected by lumbar puncture,

Table 3.7.

Constituent	Preservative	Stabilizer
Sodium	4°C or Merthiolate, Boric acid or Thymol	nil
Potassium	4°C or Merthiolate, Boric acid or Thymol	nil
Osmolality	4°C or Merthiolate, Boric acid or Thymol	nil
Urea	4°C or Merthiolate, Boric acid or Thymol	nil
Creatinine	4°C or Merthiolate or Thymol	nil
Calcium	nil	50 ml of 3 mol/l HCl
Phosphate	nil	50 ml of 3 mol/l HCl
Urate	nil	15 ml of 2 mol/l NaOH
Proteins	4°C or Merthiolate or Thymol	nil
Glucose	4°C or Merthiolate	nil
Chloride	4°C or Merthiolate, Boric acid or Thymol	nil
Oxalate	nil	50 ml or 3 mol/l HCl
Hydroxymeth-oxymandelic acid	nil	50 ml of 3 mol/l HCl
5-Hydroxyindole acetic acid	nil	50 ml of 3 mol/l HCl
Amylase	4°C or Merthiolate or Thymol	nil

is generally analysed for only a few constituents by the clinical chemistry laboratory. The main problem with this fluid is contamination with blood. The levels of proteins in plasma and cerebrospinal fluid are very different (Table 3.8).

Table 3.8.

Constituent	Units	Plasma	Cerebrospinal fluid
Proteins	g/l	70	0.3
Immunoglobulin G	g/l	10	0.035
Immunoglobulin M	g/l	1.5	0.0002
Immunoglobulin A	g/l	2.1	0.001
Albumin	g/l	40	0.2

Contamination of fluid with only a small quantity of blood will therefore invalidate analyses of all types of proteins.

3.6   Faeces collection

Faeces are rarely collected for clinical chemistry analyses except for faecal fat assays. Collections are usually performed for fixed time periods of three or five days. It is essential to ensure that collection is complete and no faeces passed are lost. The specimen, since generally weighed in the clinical laboratory prior to analysis, should not be contaminated with urine. Where more complex studies are being performed, these usually being carried out in specialist units, faecal markers corresponding to the start and finish of the experimental period have been used, including charcoal, carmine and gentian violet; chromium sesquioxide may be taken with each meal and the amount excreted determined by the laboratory, faecal output being assessed in relation to the amount of chromium sesquioxide passed.

3.7   Transport of specimens and stability

It is good policy to ensure that blood specimens are transported as soon as possible to the clinical laboratory for separation of the plasma or serum for analysis or for storage prior to analysis. This is particularly important for those constituents which are present in erythrocytes and will leak out on storage when the glucose present has been utilized and for unstable constituents such as the hormones mentioned earlier in this chapter.

Specimens for blood pH and gas analysis must also be transported quickly to the laboratory on ice because delay of more than 20 minutes causes Po_2 levels to change significantly if the specimen is at 4°C or room temperature and such changes also take place at 0°C in 30 minutes. pH and Pco_2 levels are rather more stable and do not change significantly for at least 30 minutes, even at room temperature. Many clinical laboratories, probably incorrectly, analyse serum or plasma specimens for glucose without preservative, generally fluoride, being present. The deterioration seen in non-preserved specimens varies depending on a large number of factors; typical results are shown in Fig. 3.2. Glucose metabolism is greater in specimens from neonates and no preservative truly prevents all loss; it has therefore been recommended that such specimens should be handled promptly and transported on ice. Cerebrospinal fluid specimens submitted for glucose analysis also require preservation with fluoride.

Certain other constituents undergo rapid deterioration. For example, serum acid phosphatase activity is unstable except at acid pH. Blood specimens must be transported quickly to the laboratory, the serum separated and the pH adjusted by addition of acid.

It is inappropriate in this text to document in more detail the stability of correctly collected specimens or the resultant serum or plasma. A compilation of the data available in the literature has been provided by Wilding, Zilva and Wilde (*see* Further reading[7]).

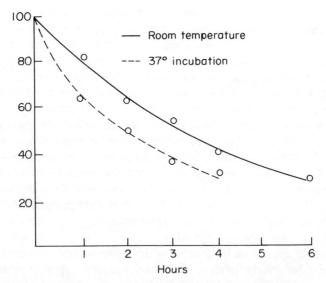

Fig. 3.2. Losses in blood glucose concentration in a specimen collected in lithium heparin without preservative. From Craig A. and Leonard P.J. (1978) In Williams D.L., Nunn R. and Marks V. Eds. *Scientific Foundations of Clinical Biochemistry,* vol. 1 (with permission from William Heinemann, London).

The transport of specimens from one hospital to another or one clinical laboratory to another is subject to regulation or legislation, in many countries. It must be emphasized that it is always appropriate for clinical laboratory staff to arrange the transport of specimens since they are aware of up-to-date local circumstances.

3.8 Separation of serum or plasma

Because of the effects of storage of whole blood on certain constituents and the requirement for serum or plasma to be used in most currently available instrumentation available for performing clinical chemistry tests nearer the patient (*see* Chapter 4), serum or plasma is sometimes separated from cells in the ward or clinic. The separation of plasma from heparinized blood by centrifugation has a major difficulty (*see* Further reading[2]). If the specimen is not centrifuged at a high enough force (3000 g) for sufficient time (15 minutes), then platelets will not be removed from the plasma. Analysis of plasma which has not been so centrifuged will give high values for lactate dehydrogenase if the analytical method has conditions which cause lysis of the platelets still present. Other analytes, including urate and alkaline phosphatase, may also be affected by the presence of platelets. Similar results have also been noted with other anticoagulants.

3.9 Summary

An analytical result cannot be of high quality unless the specimen submitted for analysis is also of high quality. Collection of specimens is generally considered straightforward but has many potential pitfalls. It must be ensured that all specimens are collected at the right time without trauma from the correctly identified patients from the appropriate site, without contamination, placed in the correct container with appropriate anticoagulant, preservative or stabilizer, transported to the clinical laboratory under the right conditions in a timeous manner and stored until analysis in a manner which prevents degradation.

Further reading

1   Calam R.R. & Cooper M.H. (1982) Recommended 'order of draw' for collecting blood specimens into additive-

containing tubes. *Clinical Chemistry,* **28,** 1399.

2   Duggan P.F., Hurly T. & Martin M. (1985) Centrifugation speeds and the removal of platelets from heparinized plasma. *Clinical Chemistry,* **31,** 1082.

3   Fraser C.G. (1985) Urine analysis: current performance and strategies for improvement. *British Medical Journal,* **291,** 321.

4   Shephard M.D.S. & Mazzachi R.D. (1983) The collection, preservation, storage and stability of urine specimens for routine clinical biochemical analysis. *The Clinical Biochemist Reviews,* **4,** 61.

5   Slockbower J.M. & Blumenfeld T.A. (1983) *Collection and Handling of Laboratory Specimens: A Practical Guide.* Lipincott, Philadelphia.

6   Statland B.E., Bokelund H. & Winkel P. (1974) Factors contributing to intraindividual variation of serum constituents: 4. Effects of posture and tourniquet application on variation of serum constituents in healthy subjects. *Clinical Chemistry,* **20,** 1513.

7   Wilding P., Zilva J.F. & Wilde C.E. (1977) Transport of specimens for clinical chemistry analysis. *Annals of Clinical Biochemistry,* **14,** 301.

Chapter 4

Analytical Concepts

4.1 Introduction

In order to be able to interpret correctly the numerical clinical laboratory test result, it is necessary to have a basic knowledge of some analytical concepts.

Traditionally clinical staff members do not perform analyses themselves, except perhaps for urine testing using reagent pad dip-sticks and other such simple procedures. However, many small analytical systems are now available which are alleged to be suitable for providing test results close to the patient. Moreover, reagent kit sets can be purchased for almost any clinical laboratory test; these provide all necessary chemicals and instructions and are often thought to be simple and straightforward to use. It is to be expected, therefore, that many of the users of clinical laboratory test results will also become providers. Good results can only come about through good analytical practice and this is a further reason, in this text, to deal with some analytical concepts.

4.2 Analytical terminology

The performance of any analytical method can be described by its *performance characteristics*. There are two groups of characteristics. *Practicability characteristics* are mainly of interest to laboratory managers and staff and include the following: type of specimen; volume required; reagents required; laboratory facilities needed; safety; skills required; necessary training; additional materials required.

More important from the interpretation of results point of

view are the *reliability characteristics* which include: analytical range; imprecision; inaccuracy; detection limit; interference; specificity.

The International Federation of Clinical Chemistry, through the Expert Panel on Nomenclature and Principles of Quality Control in Clinical Chemistry, has provided firm definitions for these characteristics (*see* Further reading[3]).

Analytical range is the range of concentration (or other quantity) in the specimen over which the method is applicable without modification.

Imprecision is the standard deviation or coefficient of variation of the results in a set of replicate measurements.

Inaccuracy is the numerical difference between the mean of a set of replicate measurements and the true value (the correct concentration or other quantity).

Detection limit is the smallest single result which (with a stated probability) can be distinguished from a true blank.

Interference is the effect of a component which does not by itself produce a reading on the accuracy of measurement of an other component.

Specificity is the ability of a method to determine solely the component(s) it purports to measure.

Although many other terms are used in clinical laboratory practice, there is no doubt that communication between clinical laboratory staff themselves and, more importantly, between clinical and laboratory staff would be enhanced by all using the same semantics.

4.3   Imprecision and inaccuracy

It is relatively easy to understand the concepts of analytical range, detection limit, interference and specificity. Confusion does arise however with the concepts of imprecision and inaccuracy.

These concepts can be visualized using the analogy of the series of diagrams shown in Fig. 4.1. If a fisherman can cast all his flies nearly always in the same spot, he has low imprecision (a) but, if he always misses the fish, he has inaccuracy. In contrast, if the fisherman casts his flies around the fish but not in a close group, he has higher imprecision but is generally near the fish and therefore has low inaccuracy (b). If the ideal occurs, the fisherman casts all his flies in a group as close as possible to the fish and he achieves low imprecision and inaccuracy (c).

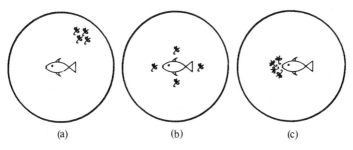

   (a)   (b)   (c)

Fig. 4.1. Diagrammatic representation of the concepts of imprecision and inaccuracy.

Imprecision

If an analyst took a single specimen of plasma and undertook 20 tests for glucose, the results would not all be exactly the same. Results would be, for example (mmol/l):

4.3	4.4	4.2	4.3
4.4	4.5	4.5	4.4
4.3	4.7	4.4	4.6
4.1	4.6	4.5	4.3
4.5	4.6	4.3	4.2

The results are not identical because of random variation

which is termed imprecision. This variation arises from sources such as the analyst filling the pipette with slightly different amounts of specimen, adding different volumes of reagent to each, incubating the assay mixtures for slightly different times and setting the spectrophotometer slightly differently each time. Imprecision is inherent in all analytical methods. It can be minimized by careful selection of method and attention to all aspects of technique but cannot be avoided.

If the results are displayed diagrammatically, a frequency histogram as shown in Fig. 4.2 is obtained. It can be seen that the distribution approximates to a smooth bell shaped curve. This is termed a Gaussian distribution. Random errors have this type of distribution, in contrast to biological variation which does not necessarily have such symmetry.

In order to delineate the Gaussian distribution characteristics, *parametric* statistics can be used because derivation of

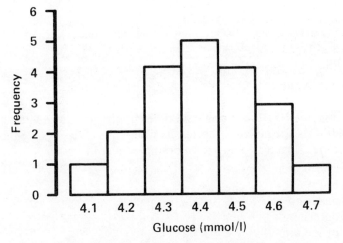

Fig. 4.2.   Frequency histogram of 20 replicate glucose analysis.

certain parameters can be simply calculated which describe the distribution in a type of shorthand.

The requirements are for, firstly, an assessment of the *central tendency*. This is usually taken as the *mean,* that is:

$$\frac{\text{the sum of all the numbers}}{\text{the number of numbers}} = \frac{\Sigma x}{n} = \bar{x}$$

Other assessments of the central tendency, the *mode* (the most common number) and the *median* (the middle number), are in fact the same as the mean for a Gaussian distribution.

Secondly, an assessment of the *dispersion* of the distribution is needed. The simplest measure is the *range:* the difference between the lowest and highest numbers. A more useful measure is the *standard deviation* (SD) which can be calculated or computed using a number of formulae usually:

$$SD = \sqrt{\frac{\Sigma(\bar{x}-x)^2}{n-1}}$$

The standard deviation has the property that if the mean ± 1 SD are taken, the central 67% of the distribution is selected and the mean ± 2 SD and mean ± 3 SD encompass 95 and 99.7% respectively. This is shown in Fig. 4.3.

The standard deviation can be expressed as a percentage of the mean value and this is termed the *coefficient of variation:*

$$CV = \frac{SD}{\bar{x}} \times 100\%$$

The CV is used a great deal in laboratory medicine and is useful when thinking about SD at different levels. For example, if plasma glucose and serum sodium analyses both had imprecision (1 SD) of 1 mmol/l, then, since this was determined at a glucose level of 5.0 mmol/l and a sodium level of 150 mmol/l, the CV of glucose assays is $1.0/5.0 \times 100 = 20\%$ but the CV of sodium assays is $1.0/150 \times 100 = 0.7\%$.

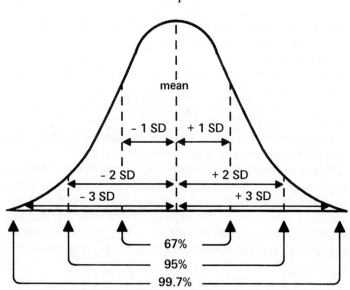

Fig. 4.3.   Characteristics of the Gaussian distribution.

For the replicate glucose data detailed above, the mean is 4.4 mmol/l and the SD is 0.16 mmol/l; the CV is therefore 3.6%.

Inaccuracy

If the true value of the specimen analysed 20 times was indeed 4.4 mmol/l then the method would have no inaccuracy. If the mean value was different, however, the method would have inaccuracy or *bias*.

Inaccuracy is due to *systematic* variation. This variation arises from sources such as using a pipette which does not deliver the correct volume of specimen or reagents, incubation in a water bath which is not the correct temperature, using a spectrophotometer which is not set at the correct wavelength, using a standard which has not actually got the value assigned.

Inaccuracy may be *constant* (the analytical results are inaccurate by the same amount at all levels) or *proportional* (the analytical results are inaccurate by the same relative amount at different levels). Inaccuracy of both types may occur simultaneously and, in addition, both types of inaccuracy may be positive or negative.

Some of the possible situations are shown in Fig. 4.4 where the found values (y-axis) are plotted against the true values (x-axis). When there is constant or proportional inaccuracy, the found results will not be equal to the true value. When constant and proportional bias are both present and are of different sign the true value is obtained, but only at one level!

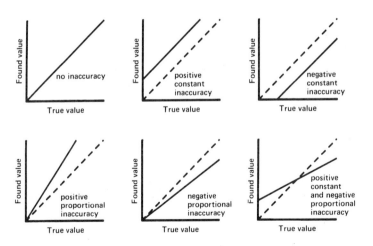

Fig. 4.4. Various situations demonstrating positive and negative constant and proportional inaccuracy.

4.4   Imprecision data

As a guide, the median imprecision obtained in 1984 for serum constituents by laboratories in the United Kingdom is shown in Table 4.1 but it must be remembered that half of the laboratories will achieve lower imprecisions than those quoted and half higher (*see* Further reading[10]). These data have been generated from an interlaboratory quality assurance survey in which many laboratories analysed, over a six month period, a series of specimens which were partly interrelated. Less data are available on urinary analytes but an Australian group (*see* Further reading[9]) have provided median laboratory performance data over a recent three year period in the readily accessible literature. The data from 1983 are shown in Table 4.2.

It is stressed that there is no rule of thumb which applies to the imprecision of tests and that they are very method and laboratory dependent. In the Australasian urine programme, for example, for urinary urea assays, the median laboratory imprecisions (1 SD) for different methods were:

diacetyl monoxime methods   11.8 mmol/l
urease/colorimetry   22.0 mmol/l
urease/conductivity   10.2 mmol/l

The overall median imprecision achieved was 13.8 mmol/l but the top 10% of laboratories could attain SD of 4.8 mmol/l or less. All clinical laboratories should provide the users with the fullest information on the imprecision achieved.

It is of interest that, for some analytes in serum and urine, the imprecisions for both these biological fluids are similar, for example:

sodium   serum SD 1.3 mmol/l
          urine SD 1.4 mmol/l

chloride serum SD 1.5 mmol/l
          urine SD 1.6 mmol/l

Table 4.1. Median imprecision achieved for serum constituents in 1984 by British laboratories.

Serum constituent	Units	Imprecision (1 SD)
Albumin	g/l	1.1
Bicarbonate	mmol/l	0.9
Bilirubin	μmol/l	2.6
Calcium	mmol/l	0.055
Chloride	mmol/l	1.5
Cholesterol	mmol/l	0.14
Creatinine	μmol/l	7.2
Glucose	mmol/l	0.19
Iron	μmol/l	1.6
Total iron binding capacity	μmol/l	4.3
Lithium	mmol/l	0.045
Magnesium	mmol/l	0.050
Osmolality	mmol/kg	3.9
Phosphate	mmol/l	0.04
Potassium	mmol/l	0.07
Proteins	g/l	1.5
Sodium	mmol/l	1.3
Triglycerides	mmol/l	0.075
Urea	mmol/l	0.33
Urate	mmol/l	0.014
Acid phosphatase	U/l	1.8
Alanine aminotransferase	U/l	4.5
Alkaline phosphatase	U/l	7.0
Amylase	U/l	21
Aspartate aminotransferase	U/l	3.6
Creatine kinase	U/l	18
Gamma-glutamyltransferase	U/l	4.0
Hydroxybutyrate dehydrogenase	U/l	18
Lactate dehydrogenase	U/l	24

In contrast, for other analytes, the imprecision of urinary analyses looks poorer than that obtained for analyses of the

Table 4.2. Median imprecision achieved for some urinary constituents in 1983 by Australian laboratories.

Urine constituent	Units	Imprecision (1 SD)
Sodium	mmol/l	1.4
Potassium	mmol/l	1.4
Osmolality	mmol/kg	5.8
Urea	mmol/l	13.8
Creatinine	mmol/l	0.44
Calcium	mmol/l	0.09
Phosphate	mmol/l	1.05
Urate	mmol/l	0.48
Proteins	g/l	0.11
Glucose	mmol/l	0.4
Chloride	mmol/l	1.6
Oxalate	mmol/l	0.05
Hydroxymethoxymandelic acid	μmol/l	13.8
5-Hydroxyindoleacetic acid	μmol/l	13.3

same analyte in serum, for example:

urea	serum	SD	0.33 mmol/l
	urine	SD	13.8 mmol/l
calcium	serum	SD	0.055 mmol/l
	urine	SD	0.09 mmol/l

These apparent differences are certainly in part due to the levels of the constituents in the two fluids and use of the CV statistic in such cases might therefore be helpful. These can be calculated and give:

urea	serum	CV	3.2%
	urine	CV	5.6%
calcium	serum	CV	2.1%
	urine	CV	3.7%

The imprecisions for the urinary analyses do appear to be larger and an important principle can be drawn from these data. Urinary assays often require an extra procedural step involving dilution of the specimen prior to analyses. All steps involve random errors and these errors are additive. In fact it is simple to calculate errors in that the *variances* (SD^2) are added. For example, if the analytical imprecision (SD) for urea assays was 0.33 mmol/l and the random error in diluting the urine specimens (SD) was 0.2 mmol/l, the total imprecision could be calculated as follows:

$$SD^2\,_{total} = SD^2\,_{analytical} + SD^2\,_{dilution}$$
$$SD_{total} = \sqrt{SD^2\,_{analytical} + SD^2\,_{dilution}}$$
$$= \sqrt{(0.33)^2 + (0.2)^2}$$
$$= \sqrt{0.1489} = 0.39 \text{ mmol/l}$$

4.5 Uses of imprecision data

Knowledge of imprecision data does assist in the interpretation of numerical clinical laboratory test results.

Firstly, most laboratories report results as single numbers, for example: plasma glucose: 4.4 mmol/l. However, since the imprecision of glucose assays is (for a particular laboratory) 1 SD = 0.2 mmol/l, it is apparent from the previous section that this single result actually has: a 67% chance of lying between 4.4±0.2, i.e. 4.2 and 4.6 mmol/l, a 95% chance of lying between 4.4±0.4, i.e. 4.0 and 4.8 mmol/l and a 99.7% chance of lying between 4.4±0.6, i.e. 3.8 and 5.0 mmol/l.

All single results do have this possible range of values and this is particularly important to remember when comparing results with reference values. A serum sodium of 146 mmol/l, when naively compared to an upper reference limit of 145 mmol/l would usually be called 'high' or 'abnormal'. Because the imprecision is 1 mmol/l, then the result lies (with the usually applied tolerance limits of 95%) between 144 and 148 mmol/l and could therefore be within the reference interval. Similarly, a serum sodium of 144 mmol/l could be 'abnormal' or, a better description, greater than the upper reference limit.

Secondly, imprecision data can provide an assessment of whether an *analytically* significant change has occurred in two results from specimens obtained sequentially from an individual. If two results differ by more than 2.8 SD, there is a 95% chance that the difference is analytically significant. As one example, the results shown in Table 4.3 were obtained on two consecutive days on a 68-year-old woman admitted to the coronary care unit with chest pain. The differences and imprecisions of the tests are also shown.

All the constituent levels change numerically but only the changes marked with an asterisk are *analytically* significant.

These two uses of imprecision data are advocated in a number of clinical laboratory texts. However, it is vital to recognize that, in addition to analytical variation, biological variation must be taken into account in the interpretation of single numerical results and in the assessment of the significance of changes in serial results from an individual. This subject is dealt with in greater depth in Chapter 6.

In addition, data on imprecision should be remembered when considering the value of the number of significant figures used in reporting test results. Many automated analysers used in clinical laboratories and computer based data handling and reporting systems do lead to results with many 'significant' figures being produced and reported. This should not be done (since one of the means whereby the imprecision of a test can be communicated to users is by using the correct number of significant figures) but it does occur. As an example, consider the way two laboratories, who have identical imprecision of CV $-$ 5%, report the results of paediatric bilirubins assay on

Table 4.3.

Constituent	Units	Day 1	Day 2	Difference	Imprecision (SD)
Sodium	mmol/l	135	146	11*	1.3
Potassium	mmol/l	4.4	4.9	0.5*	0.07
Chloride	mmol/l	101	106	5*	1.5
Bicarbonate	mmol/l	20	18	2	0.9
Urea	mmol/l	37.6	37.7	0.1	0.33
Creatinine	μmol/l	212	247	35*	7.2
Calcium	mmol/l	2.14	2.43	0.29*	0.055
Albumin	g/l	31	37	6*	1.1
Phosphate	mmol/l	1.48	1.90	0.42*	0.04
Alkaline phosphatase	U/l	136	145	9	7.0
Bilirubins	μmol/l	12	18	6	2.6
Proteins	g/l	56	64	8*	1.5

a series of specimens.

Laboratory 1	Laboratory 2
341.2	340
289.3	290
267.8	270
64.6	60
193.2	190

The results reported by laboratory 1, which uses an automatic data handling system programmed by a nonlaboratory-orientated individual, do give an impression of having low imprecision. On the other hand, the results reported by laboratory 2 in numerical increments of 10 do give a realistic indicator of the imprecision actually achieved.

4.6   Inaccuracy

As for imprecision, the inaccuracy obtained by laboratories is different because of the variety of methods and techniques used, type of calibrator used, mode of calibration and other factors. This performance characteristic is much more difficult to quantitate and often laboratories consider inaccuracy to be of little importance because it is said to be taken into account in the reference values generated by the particular laboratory. This is certainly one good reason why reference values are not transferable from laboratory to laboratory and why reference values from textbooks and other material should not be used to aid in the interpretation of the results of clinical laboratory tests. This subject is dealt with in detail in Chapter 5.

Laboratory results should have no inaccuracy. If this ideal were achieved, then results from different laboratories would be more comparable; results would be more compatible over a time period because changes in laboratory equipment, methods and techniques would not lead to changes in inaccuracy, reference values would be more comparable between laboratories and rigid numerical criteria for the interpretation of results and initiation of clinical action could be better applied.

4.7 Other performance characteristics

The analytical range and the detection limit are mainly of interest to laboratory staff. The ramifications for interpretation of laboratory results are that results outside the range are often reported as 'less than' or 'more than' certain values and results lower than the detection limit are often reported as 'less than' that value. When the initial result is higher than the upper limit of the range, it is usual laboratory policy to dilute and reanalyse the specimen. As discussed previously, this additional dilution procedure will lead to greater imprecision and, as a general rule, the imprecision of very high results will be higher than that at the reference limits and at clinical decision making levels. Laboratories sometimes prepare 'precision profiles' showing the relationship between imprecision and constituent level; this is usually done in detail only for hormone assays where the type of immunoassay conventionally used in laboratories leads to greater imprecision at both high and low levels (*see* Further reading[7]).

The detection limit of certain tests can, on occasion, limit their clinical usefulness. For example, some would suggest that a good strategy to investigate patients with thyrometabolic disease would be to measure serum thyrotrophin (TSH) as an initial test. Those with low TSH levels would be further investigated for hyperthyroidism. Unfortunately, most traditional assays for serum TSH have a detection limit which is at a level that does not allow clear discrimination between euthyroid and hyperthyroid subjects. Newer assays with lower detection limits may change this situation.

The problems associated with interferences and specificity of tests have already been dealt with in Chapters 2 and 3. Problems arise from the patient, where the previous intake of food and drink and *in vitro* effects of drugs may cause analytical problems. The specimen itself, through collection contamination, inappropriate anticoagulation or preservation, haemolysis, and the presence due to disease of high levels of a constituent usually present in low concentrations may cause difficulties in test result interpretation. Again it is worthy of note that different laboratory methods are interfered with by different substances or by the same compound to different extents and also that they may have different specificities. The advice of the laboratory should always be sought if such problems are suspected.

4.8 Clinical chemistry close to the patient

As outlined in Chapter 1, the process by which clinicians obtain numerical results from a laboratory is complex; different types of staff are involved and there are sources of real or potential error at each stage in the process. Many now hold the view that technology has advanced to such an extent that a number of tests can now be performed close to the patient and certain of the sources of error eliminated (*see* Further reading[8]). Moreover, other advantages are that (i) the turnaround times between specimen collection and availability of results are minimized, (ii) tests may be performed at the times considered necessary rather than as dictated by the laboratory, (iii) clinically essential tests may be frequently performed, (iv) treatment may be rapidly initiated or modified and (v) costs associated with transport and purchase of large centralized laboratory equipment may be saved.

The performance of clinical biochemistry laboratory tests close to the patient does have disadvantages. The vast majority of objective studies on the analytical performance achieved in wards and clinics show that the standards attained are worse than those reached in laboratories. The reagents used in most analytical systems suitable for use in such situations are expensive. The requirement to purchase many small analytical systems for a large number of areas in even a medium-sized hospital means that significant capital is likely to be expended. Many clinicians are very unaware of the sources of error involved in patient preparation and specimen collection; it is often very difficult to detect these errors when only a single test result is available. Most potential users of the analytical systems have little experience in analysis, instrument maintenance and fault-finding or quality control. Instrumentation and reagents, once purchased, may be used so infrequently that satisfactory performance characteristics cannot be achieved when a result is really required urgently and the analytical technique is attempted for the first time in a long period. The need to separate serum or plasma from cells prior to analysis is a major problem with most current methodology. The analytical methodology may be rather different to that used in the central laboratory leading to severe problems of interpretation if results are generated on a single patient using more than one technique.

At present, it is theoretically possible to perform a wide range of analyses in wards and clinics, principally using technology based on ion-selective electrodes, dry reagent systems and reflectance meters with reagent dip-sticks. Recent advances include the small scale introduction of immunoassay techniques and bio-sensors. Analyses studied include those shown in Table 4.4.

Other analyses may also be performed in wards and clinics such as sweat chloride in patients suspected of having cystic fibrosis and faecal occult blood tests.

Introduction of clinical biochemistry tests closer to the patient can best be performed if the guidelines similar to those

Table 4.4.

Blood	Serum/plasma	Urine
gases	glucose	pH
glucose	sodium	protein
urea	potassium	glucose
lactate	urea	ketones
	therapeutic drugs	bilirubin
	bilirubins (in neonates)	nitrite
	osmolality	urobilinogen
	creatine kinase	vitamin C
	thyroxine	specific gravity
		electrolytes
		osmolality

proposed jointly by the Royal College of Pathologists, Association of Clinical Pathologists and Association of Clinical Biochemists are followed (*see* Further reading[1]); almost identical guidelines have been proposed in certain other countries. The guidelines encompass the following points:

(i)   There should be *liaison* between laboratory and clinician before instrumentation is introduced.

(ii)   *Selection* and *assessment* of methods should be performed in collaboration with the laboratory.

(iii)   All aspects of the use of the technique should comply with current *health* and *safety* legislation and practice.

(iv)   All users of the technique should be *trained, listed* as approved users and *supervised.* Good *record keeping* is essential.

(v)   Adequate *internal quality control* should be carried out and records kept. An *external quality assessment* scheme should, if possible, be used.

(vi)   *Maintenance* and dealing with *faults* should be the responsibility of the central laboratory.

(vii)   *Staff* may require to be provided from the central laboratory to meet all these guidelines.

(viii)   Continued *collaboration* between *ward* and *clinic* staffs and the *laboratory* staff is essential.

A likely future extension to the performance of clinical biochemistry tests outside the laboratory, one which has existed for some years with the analysis of urinary and blood glucose by patients with diabetes mellitus, is the growth of 'home testing' or 'self-testing' (*see* Further reading[6]). Currently most of this type of testing is initiated by the clinician and it is essential that, should this field expand, the home or self operator be made aware of certain of the more basic analytical concepts outlined in this chapter.

4.9   Assessment of analytical methods

If it is decided to perform tests outside the clinical laboratory, no matter whether the method is a traditional technique or makes use of an analyser or a reagent kit set, it is mandatory to assess objectively whether the performance characteristics are such that the method is satisfactory for its intended use.

Most evaluations are not well designed or executed (even by clinical biochemists). This has been documented by Fraser and Singer (*see* Further reading[5]). It must be realized that proper selection and evaluation of methods is not a task that should be undertaken lightly. Considerable knowledge and expertise are required for the setting up of the study, the performance of the experiments, the statistical analysis of the large amount of data generated and the interpretation of the results. It is advocated, therefore, that evaluation of new methods should be performed by experts in laboratories which have specialist interests in this facet of laboratory work. As a consequence, really new methods, instruments or kits should not be introduced outside the laboratory without considerable experience being accumulated first by the specialists.

It follows that only well tried and tested methods should be introduced outside the laboratory. In this situation, an assessment rather than a full evaluation should be undertaken and, as stated earlier, it is best if this be done in close collaboration with the laboratory. There are many published protocols for assessment and evaluation of methods. Most are written for the knowledgeable clinical chemist and are somewhat theoretical. One, however, has been specifically prepared for the relatively inexperienced by White and Fraser (*see* Further reading[14]).

Any assessment consists of six stages:

pre-evaluation assessment

familiarization

assessment

specific studies

assessment of performance

introduction to service

Pre-evaluation assessment is the selection of the method or a few methods that seem likely to be very suitable for the task to be performed. This is best done by careful documentation of the ideal with respect to:

analytes it is wished to assay

patient type being handled

type of specimens it is wished to analyse

volume of specimen available

number of assays to be done

turnaround time required from specimen collection to result availability

ideal performance characteristics

imprecision

inaccuracy

analytical range

    detection limit
    interference and specificity
  skills required
  space required
  facilities (power, water, gas) required
  ancillary equipment (pipettes, centrifuge, vials) required
  reagents required
  costs—capital and ongoing

When the ideal is very well thought out and described, it is relatively easy to prepare a check list and, from information available from the published literature, governmental sources, professional bodies, manufacturer's literature and informed colleagues, to select one to three methods, instruments or reagent kit sets which appear to fulfil the needs.

Familiarization

When the likely methods are obtained for assessment, before detailed experimental studies are performed it is essential to make sure that the analyst is familiar with the technique. This includes ensuring that:

  the method is in a suitable site
  all services, reagents and ancillary equipment are available
  the method is working more or less as expected

Assessment

Since the method has been well studied in the past, it should only be necessary, when the familiarization period is complete, to perform a short study to confirm that the performance characteristics obtained do match the data previously documented and that they are acceptable for the requirements.

The procedure is to analyse a number of specimens from patients in duplicate. At least 40 specimens should be analysed. The duplicate assays should be performed in different analytical batches since it is the between-batch imprecision that is the important characteristic. The specimens should be selected carefully to give a wide range of analyte levels and to include potential interfering substances such as bilirubins, haemoglobin and lipaemia.

The specimens should also be analysed in duplicate by a comparative method. This method would ideally have small imprecision, no inaccuracy and a wide analytical range. However, this ideal is rarely achievable and it would be more usual to analyse the specimens by the method used every day in the clinical laboratory. A wealth of information on the performance characteristics of such a method should at least be available.

When the experimental work is completed, one result from the new method is plotted against the comparative method result for the same specimen on a graph. The new method results are always plotted on the y-axis and the comparative method results are plotted on the x-axis. The mean of the duplicate pairs is not used because this lowers the imprecision (by $\sqrt{n}$, where n is the number of replicates; in this case the imprecision would be improved 1.4 times).

The graph should then be examined. By visual inspection (since statistical methods are complex) it should be possible to assess the linear range of the method and whether any outliers are present. Outliers are results which do not lie in the main cluster of results. Outliers should not merely be discarded but they should not be included in further calculations. Inspection of the duplicates should be performed to assess whether gross errors such as those due to specimen mix-up or omission of a crucial reagent has occurred. Moreover, outliers might give a clue to the possibility of drug interference or specimen problems such as could arise from the presence of icterus, haemolysis or lipaemia. The data should then be treated statistically by linear regression analysis. The statistics minimally required are:

the regression equation in the form $y = mx \pm b$

the correlation coefficient-r

the t statistic

The equation shows the systematic errors. The slope of the line (m) shows the proportional error which is called positive if m is greater than 1 and negative if m is less than 1. The intercept (b) shows the constant error which is called positive if b is positive and negative if b is negative.

The correlation coefficient estimates the degree of association between the results of new and comparative methods. The closer r is to 1, the greater the degree of association.

The t statistic is used to assess the probability that the means of the results obtained by new and comparative methods are the same. The t value obtained is compared with the critical values to t at various probability levels in t-tables found in statistical texts (*see* Further reading[11]).

An example of the type of graph obtained and the statistics generated from the data is shown in Fig. 4.5.

The imprecisions of new and comparative methods can easily be calculated by taking the differences between the pairs of results obtained by the same method, squaring each difference, adding up all the squares, dividing by twice the number of pairs of results and taking the square root. That is:

$$
\begin{aligned}
SD &= \sqrt{\frac{\Sigma(\text{difference between the pairs})^2}{2 \times \text{number of pairs}}} \\
&= \sqrt{\frac{\Sigma d^2}{2N}}
\end{aligned}
$$

The mean ($\bar{x}$) is calculated and the CV derived from the

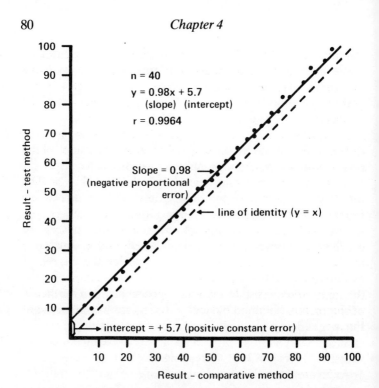

Fig. 4.5. Example of graph obtained from linear regression analysis commonly used in assessment and comparison of methods.

formula:

$$CV = \frac{SD}{\bar{x}} \times 100$$

It can be determined if the imprecision of one method is inferior or superior to the other by calculation of the F statistic. F is calculated:

$$F = \frac{\text{first } SD^2}{\text{second } SD^2}$$

and F tables in statistical texts consulted. If F is greater than the critical value of F for n-1 degrees of freedom for numerator and denominator, then the imprecision of one method is significantly worse than the imprecision of the other ($P \geq 0.05$ tables) or highly significantly different ($P \geq 0.01$ tables).

It may be advantageous to calculate the imprecision at different constituent levels by, for example, grouping the results into low, medium and high levels.

It is stressed that the statistical manipulations described here are very simple to perform. The text by Swinscow (*see* Further reading[11]) is an excellent simple introductory text which will demonstrate amply that statistics applied to medicine and laboratory work is not a difficult obscure subject to master. However, the use of statistical techniques in evaluation and assessment work does have some pitfalls for the uninitiated and the unwary; a good summary of these problems has been provided by Westgard and Hunt (*see* Further reading[12]).

Specific studies

Each assessment is unique. Consequently, specific experiments for each assessment may have to be designed and executed in order to be able to reach a decision on the usefulness or otherwise of the method. An example might be that it is wished to perform potassium assays on serum, plasma and urine using a single instrument. It would be necessary to investigate the effect of the anticoagulant on the performance characteristics. It would also be necessary to assess the performance of the method with urine specimens as well as serum because the range of levels in the two types of fluid are very different (the instrument would probably have special settings for each fluid type) and because the compositions of serum and urine specimens are far from identical.

Assessment of performance

It is difficult to decide whether a method is acceptable. If the comparative method has no inaccuracy, the new method should have

the slope (m), close to 1

the intercept (b), close to 0

the correlation coefficient (r), close to 1

no significant difference between the means of new and comparative methods (by the *t* test).

Ideally, the method should not have interferences and should be specific.

Ideally, the imprecision should attain the standards based upon biological variation data (*see* Chapter 6) and the desirable CV for some of the serum constituents analysed in wards and/or clinics are as follows:

Sodium:	0.4%	Urea:	6.2%
Potassium:	2.2%	Glucose:	2.2%
Calcium:	0.9%	Creatinine:	2.2%

The fascinating subject of the desirable standards of performance has been extensively reviewed recently (*see* Further reading[4]).

Introduction to service

If the method is judged objectively to be acceptable then, before specimens from patients are actually analysed, it is necessary to ensure the following:

staff training is complete

the work environment is suitable and safe

reference values are available (*see* Chapter 5)

reagents and consumables have been purchased

preparation of instructions for use

preparation of maintenance schedule if an instrument is
  being used
preparation of forms or sheets to record and/or report the
  analytical results
A further necessary prerequisite to the introduction of a
method to service is the setting up of comprehensive quality
control procedures.

4.10   Quality control and assessment

All methods both within and outside clinical chemistry laboratories should be subject to internal quality assessment
procedures to monitor ongoing performance and to ensure
that the standard of performance achieved during the assessment period is maintained.

The subject of quality control and assessment is very broad
(*see* Further reading[2]) and most large laboratories have a
fulltime member of staff employed as quality control officer.

Traditionally, quality control is performed using the
reference sample technique. This is based upon the premise
that effects on the results of analyses of specimens from
patients are reflected in the analytical results generated on
analysis of the same one (or more) specimens in each analytical batch. These control specimens are sometimes generated
from pools of biological material; aliquots are stored frozen
and one thawed and analysed along with each batch. This type
of material, although cheap and very similar in nature to
specimens from patients, is not recommended because of the
very real biological hazards which exist, notably that of
hepatitis. It is recommended that commercially available
freeze-dried or liquid material, preferably of human origin, be
purchased in large batches, stored appropriately, recon-
stituted as directed if required and analysed in each batch. The
material used should be chosen very carefully particularly

with respect to the level of constituents. A level at or near the point at which clinical decisions are made is ideal. It may be desirable to analyse more than one material with different levels in each batch.

Prior to using the quality control material, it is analysed 20 times, 20 being a compromise between gaining a good estimate of the characteristics of the assay and the control material and the time, effort and cost of replicate analyses. The mean and SD are then calculated after a graph has been drawn to check for stability; a graph of the values obtained on the 20 days (y-axis) against time (x-axis) should be parallel to the x-axis. The simplest criteria for ongoing use of this material are:

(i) if the results of analyses of the material are within x±2SD, the analytical batch is acceptable and the patient's results can be used for clinical purposes with confidence,

(ii) if the results of analysis of the material are outside x±3SD, the analytical batch is unacceptable, the patient's results should not be used for clinical care and steps instituted to find the sources of the problems and rectify these, and

(iii) if the results of analysis of the material are between x±2SD and x±3SD, the analytical batch is acceptable but it may be that the method is slipping out of control and attention should be paid to the factors that are known to influence the method.

There are many ways that can be used to aid in the monitoring of the analytical results obtained on the quality control material. An often used graphic technique is the Levey–Jennings plot. A graph is set up with time on the x-axis and value on the y-axis with horizontal lines at the mean, ±3SD (action limits) and ±2SD (warning limits). Each result is plotted on the graph and results can easily be assessed visually. An example is shown in Fig. 4.6. This quality control material for serum glucose analyses had, on prior replicate

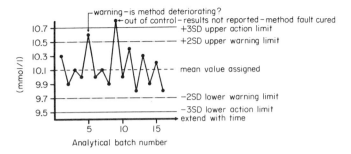

Fig. 4.6. Example of a Levey–Jennings quality control chart.

analyses 20 times, a mean value assigned as 10.1 mmol/l and SD of 0.2 mmol/l.

This method of quality control has some disadvantages. The simple ±2SD and ±3SD limits are statistically naive and this has been documented in detail by Westgard and his associates (*see* Further reading[13]), the material is expensive and may require reconstitution and the material may not mimic truly specimens from patients.

Other methods of quality control are of great value and include the following techniques.

Performance of analyses in replicate allows assessment of gross errors. Criteria can be set for acceptance or rejection of analytical batches, or for individual specimens, for example, if duplicate results differed by less than 5% the analyses could be classed as acceptable, more than 5% but less than 10% worthy of concern about methodological aspects and more than 10% classed as unacceptable. It is important to recognize that performing analyses in replicate and taking the means of the sets of data does improve the assay; the imprecision is improved $\sqrt{n}$-fold, n being the number of replicates, and therefore duplicate analyses improve imprecision by 1.4 times and triplicate analyses by 1.7 times. A possibly useful strategy to adopt for analyses done closer to the patient is to leave one specimen analysed by an operator for the next analyst to retest, provided the analyte is stable.

The clinician has an important role to play in analytical quality control. When an analytical result does not appear to fit in with either clinical impression or other analytical data, it should not simply be neglected but enquiry made as to possible sources of error. As a minimum requirement, the test ought to be repeated on a new specimen and ideally on the original specimen also.

Quality control should extend to reagents, making sure that none have expired and that they are stored correctly; to instruments, ensuring that correct maintenance has been performed, to ancillary equipment such as pipettes and dilutors (correct volumes being reproducibly delivered); centrifuges (adequate forces being achieved); water-baths (correct temperatures being achieved and maintained) and to specimens (*see* Chapters 2 and 3), only those correctly collected from adequately prepared patients being analysed. Monitoring of instrumental settings is also a useful means of quality control since, with certain techniques, the need to change the settings will indicate a deterioration in performance. Quality control should also extend to staff, only those with adequate training and skills being listed as approved users.

With many of the modern very stable analytical systems principally designed for use closer to the patient, quality control methods other than the reference sample technique are possibly of more value.

External quality assessment involves analysis of a series of specimens, aliquots of which have been sent to many laboratories. Return of results to a central organizing laboratory allows data processing of all results and regular feedback to the individual laboratory of the results obtained by other laboratories, usually classified according to methodology. Most tests commonly performed in clinical biochemistry laboratories are covered by such schemes, at least in developed countries. It is good practice for tests performed outside the central laboratory to be assessed in such schemes.

4.11 Summary

A basic knowledge of analytical nomenclature and practice is vital to the correct interpretation of laboratory results.

Knowledge of imprecision data aids interpretation of single numerical results, particularly when near to the limits of the reference intervals, and allows assessment of the analytical significance of serial results obtained from an individual patient. Different laboratory methods have different degrees of inaccuracy and this means that reference values vary from laboratory to laboratory.

With currently available technology, it is possible to perform many tests closer to the patient. This approach has advantages and disadvantages. Sensible guidelines for the adoption of this type of testing have been clearly laid down and these should be followed as far as possible.

Before any laboratory method, instrument or reagent kit set is introduced, it is necessary to perform an assessment or evaluation. This is not an easy task and a six-stage protocol involving pre-evaluation assessment, familiarization, assessment, specific studies, evaluation of experimental data and introduction to service should be carefully followed.

When any laboratory test is performed, quality control techniques must be applied. Quality control does not mean simply the occasional analysis of a specimen with known value. Quality control should also apply to reagents, instrument and ancillary equipment, environment and staff. Ideally all methods should be subject to quality assessment procedures.

Further reading

1 Anderson J.R., Linsell W.D. & Mitchell F.L. (1981) Chemical pathology on the ward. *The Lancet*, **i,** 487.

2 Bruce A.W. (1984) *Basic Quality Assurance and Quality Control in the Clinical Laboratory*. Little, Brown and Co., Boston.

3 Buttner J., Borth R., Boutwell J.H., Broughton P.M.G. & Bowyer R.C. (1979) Approved recommendation (1978) on quality control in clinical chemistry. Part 1. General principles and terminology. *Clinica chimica acta*, **98,** 129.

4 Fraser C.G. (1983) Desirable performance characteristics for clinical chemistry tests. *Advances in Clinical Chemistry*, **23,** 299.

5 Fraser C.G. & Singer R. (1985) Better laboratory evaluations of instruments and kits are required. *Clinical Chemistry*, **31,** 667.

6 Free A.H. & Free H.M. (1984) Self testing, an emerging component of clinical chemistry. *Clinical Chemistry*, **30,** 829.

7 Jeffcoate S.L. (1981) *Efficiency and Effectiveness in the Endocrine Laboratory*. Academic Press, London.

8 Marks V. & Alberti K.G.M.M. Eds. (1985) *Clinical Biochemistry Nearer the Patient*. Churchill Livingstone, Edinburgh.

9 Shephard M.D.S., Penberthy L.A. & Fraser C.G. (1984) Evolution of a national urine quality assurance programme: the Australasian experience. *Journal of Clinical Pathology*, **37,** 415.

10 Stevens J.F. & Hjelm G.C.E. (1985) Achievable standards of laboratory performance. *News Sheet, Association of Clinical Biochemists*, **262,** 14.

11 Swinscow T.D.V. (1978) *Statistics at Square One*. British Medical Association, London.

12   Westgard J.O. & Hunt M.R. (1973) Use and interpret-
     ation of common statistical tests in method comparison
     studies. *Clinical Chemistry*, **19,** 49.
13   Westgard J.O., Barry P.L. & Hunt M.R. (1981) A multi-
     rule Shewart chart for quality control in clinical chem-
     istry. *Clinical Chemistry*, **27,** 493.
14   White G.H. & Fraser C.G. (1984) The evaluation kit for
     clinical chemistry: a practical guide for the evaluation of
     methods, instruments and reagent kits. *Journal of Auto-
     matic Chemistry*, **6,** 122.

Chapter 5
Reference Values

5.1 Introduction

It is usually considered that clinical laboratory test results cannot be interpreted adequately without knowledge concerning the results found in other persons, particularly the healthy. As a result, clinical laboratory staff traditionally spend much time and effort generating 'normal' values or ranges and often expend significant resources flagging or otherwise highlighting test results which are outside these values. The users of laboratory services also spend much of their time comparing results generated on individual patients with normal values and often carefully follow up results which are considered to be 'abnormal'. In addition, many clinical texts and most clinical laboratory books, whether they concentrate on clinical or laboratory aspects of the discipline, have significant detailed information on normal values and/or their generation and entire texts are concerned with the listing of normal values and the changes which occur due to both physiological and pathological processes. Unfortunately, traditional normal values are far from satisfactory.

5.2 Problems with normal values

A number of difficulties do exist with the concept and use of normal values. A major problem is simply a semantic one because the word normal has very different meanings to different types of professional. These have been very amusingly discussed by Murphy (*see* Further reading[7]); the meanings are shown in Table 5.1, listed in decreasing order of objectivity.

Table 5.1

Meaning	Discipline	Better terminology
A probability function	Statistics	Gaussian
Most representative	Any descriptive science	Average
Commonly encountered	Any descriptive science	Habitual
Suited to survival	Genetics	Optimal
Carrying no penalty	Medicine	Harmless
Aspired to	Politics	Conventional
Most perfect	Metaphysics	Ideal

Other authors have added even further semantic uses to the list.

There is no doubt that these different meanings of the term normal have caused significant confusion because, at least for some laboratory tests, all of the meanings can be applied in manners which do make sense.

In part because the word normal is used to describe the Gaussian distribution, it has been and still is commonplace to derive normal values by applying parametric statistical techniques to data and the mean and standard deviation (SD) are derived without assessing whether the distribution is actually Gaussian or not. The mean ±2SD, which is assumed to encompass 95% of the data, is then termed the normal range of values. However, it must be realized that biological data is not necessarily distributed in a Gaussian manner and application of simple statistical techniques without prior assessment of the distribution is not good practice. For many analytes assayed by the clinical laboratory, the distribution of data derived from a population does not have a Gaussian distribution and the data is skewed, particularly usual being tailing to higher values; for example, serum alkaline phosphatase and serum bilirubins show such distributions. If the mean ±2SD range is derived from such data, then it is found that the lower limit of this range is actually less than zero. This is impossible and the facile solutions are to quote normal values as 'less than' a certain result or 'up to' a result.

This situation can be alleviated by another widely adopted strategy, that of using 'log normal' statistics where each data point (or the means of sets of data points) is (or are) taken and the logarithms of each derived, the mean ±2SD calculated from the logarithmic data and the normal range calculated by taking antilogarithms. This strategy simply ensures that the range does not encompass negative numbers. Further techniques can be applied to data which are not Gaussianly distributed, the most commonly used being to attempt to disect out normal values by graphical approaches, either simply by visual inspection or, in a more complex manner, using probability paper. Clear descriptions of these approaches are given in the widely available text of Barnett (*see* Further reading[2]), but, because they all make assumptions about the distribution characteristics of the population data, they have disadvantages and are currently considered less than ideal.

A further grave problem is the application of the concept that there is a direct link between normality and health. It is often erroneously thought that the finding of a test result within normal values can be equated with health (and therefore such results either can be ignored or provide firm evidence of the absence of disease) and that the occurrence of an abnormal result must mean that disordered structure or function is present and must be followed up to a logical conclusion.

Finally, it must be remembered that most data on normal

values is provided without adequate information on the subjects studied or the techniques used for specimen collection, analysis and data reduction and, as will be discussed in detail later, such factors have significant influence on normal values.

5.3   The reference value concept

Because of the many difficulties with normal values, Grasbeck and Saris, in 1969, introduced a new terminology, that of *reference values* (*see* Further reading[4]).

This new terminology was very quickly adopted by clinical laboratories but, unfortunately, has not yet become ubiquitously used. It must be noted that the newer term 'reference values' is not merely a replacement for the older term 'normal values'. The term reference values implies that the mode of generation of the values is known with respect to at least the following factors:

selection of subjects

assessment of the state of health

characteristics of the population, such as age and sex

specimen collection and storage

analytical technique performance characteristics

data handling technique

5.4   Further definitions

The International Federation of Clinical Chemistry, through the Expert Panel on Theory of Reference Values, has spent considerable effort over the past 15 years developing the concepts of reference values. The first paper which resulted from their work proposed a series of terms which were judged to be concise and well defined (*see* Further reading[5]). These terms are as follows:

(i)   A *reference individual* is an individual selected using defined criteria.

(ii)   A *reference population* consists of all possible reference individuals.

(iii)   A *reference sample group* is an adequate number of reference individuals selected to represent the reference population.

(iv)   A *reference value* is the value obtained by observation or measurement of a particular type of quantity on a reference individual.

(v)   A *reference distribution* is the distribution of reference values.

(vi)   A *reference limit* is derived from the reference distribution and is used for descriptive purposes.

(vii)   A *reference interval* is the interval between, and including two reference limits.

(viii)   *An observed value* is a value of a particular type of quantity, obtained by observation or measurement, to be compared with reference values, reference distributions, reference limits or reference intervals.

The terms are unambiguous and the Expert Panel suggest that universal adoption of the terminology would improve both the understanding of reference values and the interpretation of observed values (test results). The relationship between the terms is shown in Fig. 5.1.

5.5   Factors affecting reference values

Although this new terminology regarding reference values has been developed, it is highly unlikely that a single set of values can be used to interpret the results of each clinical laboratory test. This is because there are very many factors which affect individuals. These factors can be grouped in a number of ways

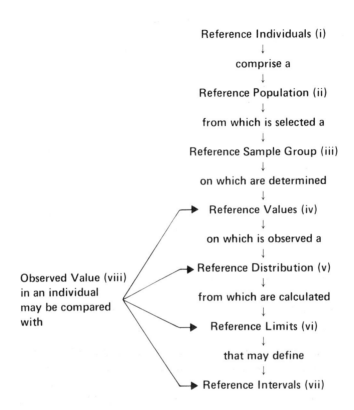

Fig. 5.1. Diagram showing the relationship between the definitions proposed by the IFCC Expert Panel on Theory of Reference Values.

and one logical approach is to divide the factors into four groups, namely, laboratory factors, endogenous factors, exogenous factors and genetic factors. These are discussed below but it must be realized that it is impossible to provide exhaustive information on all factors influencing every clinical laboratory test in this text.

5.6 Laboratory factors

Although clinical laboratories of comparable size generally offer similar repertoires of tests, the specimen collection, transport and storage and the analytical techniques adopted do vary significantly. Many of these factors affect reference values including the following, which have been discussed in detail in Chapter 3.

Specimen collection, transport and storage

The *type* of *blood specimen* collected and subsequently analysed, whether it be arterial, capillary or venous, can markedly affect reference values. For example, the criteria for individuals not having diabetes mellitus are, for specimens taken at 2 hours following a 75 g oral load in nonpregnant adults, that the venous blood glucose should be < 6.7 mmol/l and the capillary blood glucose should be < 7.8 mmol/l.

Another relevant example is that serum and plasma reference values are not identical for constituents that are present in erythrocytes in high concentrations or activities. The clotting process results in the reference values for serum potassium, phosphate, lactate dehydrogenase, hydroxybutyrate dehydrogenase and aspartate aminotransferase being higher for serum than for plasma specimens.

The usual *time delay* between the taking of specimens and their receipt and processing by the laboratory may also affect reference values. For example, the changes seen in serum as compared to plasma will be even larger as the time delay increases. Other effects also occur, for example, the serum bicarbonate level will fall with time as the CO_2 equilibrates with the low $P\text{CO}_2$ of ambient air. The time for which the tourniquet is applied as a usual procedure to facilitate the collection of venous blood will also affect laboratory results and therefore reference values, particularly for constituents that are proteins or are bound to protein in some way (in whole or part) such as serum calcium, bilirubins and cholesterol.

Analytical technique

Imprecision of laboratory techniques cannot be avoided, although it can be minimized by judicious selection of methodology and by introduction of a variety of strategies to improve laboratory performance. The magnitude of the imprecision will affect reference values. For example, if it was assumed that the mean value for serum sodium was 140 mmol/l and that the distribution of the true values was completely Gaussian and had SD = 3 mmol/l, then the reference interval (biological) which encompassed 95% of the population would be:

Mean±2SD
140 ± 6.0 mmol/l
134 to 146 mmol/l

If the imprecision was 1.0 mmol/l, then, because variance-$(SD)^2$ is additive,

the total SD $= \sqrt{1^2+3^2} = \sqrt{10} = 3.2$

and the reference interval becomes

140±6.4 mmol/l
133.6 to 146.4 mmol/l.

For an analytical technique with twice the imprecision, that is 2.0 mmol/l, then,

the total SD $= \sqrt{2^2+3^2} = \sqrt{13} = 3.6$
and the reference interval becomes

140±7.2 mmol/l
132.8 to 147.2 mmol/l

The inaccuracy of laboratory methods also will affect reference values in a manner which is proportional to the methodological bias.

5.7 Endogenous factors

Endogenous factors which affect reference values are those that are inherent to individuals and cannot be modified, at least in a major way. There are a number of these influences, which include age, sex and body mass.

In addition, biological rhythms are very important endogenous factors and these will be dealt with in detail in Chapter 6.

Age

Many constitutents assayed by the clinical laboratory do change with age. Certain analytes change in what could be described as a linear fashion, for example, the mean serum phosphate level falls in post-pubertal life up to age 65 and the mean serum creatinine rises in this manner after age 20. Others do not show such regular changes, for example, the mean serum cholesterol level rises with age until the fifth decade of life and then falls (perhaps because those with higher cholesterol levels have suffered early coronary vascular disease) and the mean serum alkaline phosphatase activity falls after the pubertal growth period, in which osteoblastic activity is high due to bone building, and then rises in later adult life. These changes in Canadian men, taken from the Sherbrooke population study, are shown in Fig. 5.2. Many changes reported in adult life are not marked, however, and there are sometimes conflicting reports in the literature.

In the elderly, significant changes occur particularly in post

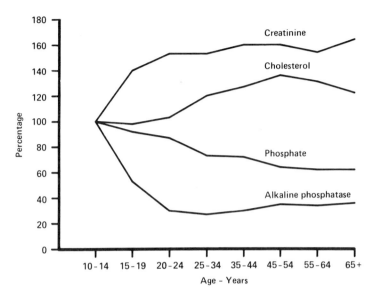

Fig. 5.2.   Changes in the serum concentrations of Canadian adult men with age; the 50th percentile is given and results expressed as percentages of the concentration or activity at 10–14 years of age. Data from the Sherbrooke study (See Further reading[4]).

menopausal women in whom serum calcium, cholesterol, phosphate, sodium, urate and urea levels rise. Indeed, from the clinical chemist's point of view particularly, postmenopausal women are very like elderly men. Hormonal responses become diminished in the elderly and, although the serum levels of many hormones do not change significantly, the concentrations of certain of the hormones assayed by the clinical laboratory are significantly affected, urinary 17-oxo- and 17-oxogenic steroids, serum testosterone (in the male), serum renin and angiotensin all decreasing with increasing age.

The changes that occur in the new born and during childhood are many and varied; these have been well documented in at least one excellent source book (*see* Further reading[6]) and they cannot be dealt with in depth in this text. When the influence of age on laboratory test results is considered, it is not always simply the chronological age that is important, although reference values are frequently stratified in this manner. Physiological age, in terms of, for example, whether the menopause or puberty has been passed, is often much more relevant.

Sex

Pre-pubertal boys and girls are biochemically similar, as are postmenopausal women and elderly men. It is during the reproductive phase of life that sex differences significantly affect test results except for the influences of muscle mass. Most effects, such as the comparatively increased concentrations or activities of the following serum constituents are due to the influences of oestrogens:

alanine aminotransferase	aldolase
aspartate aminotransferase	alkaline phosphatase
albumin	total proteins
calcium	magnesium
prolactin	growth hormone

Certain analytes have lower levels in the female of reproductive years including serum iron, ferritin, bilirubins and haemoglobin.

Body mass

A large number of serum constituents are positively correlated with body mass including:

creatine kinase	creatinine
cholesterol	triglycerides
urate	triiodothyronine

Some are negatively correlated, including serum iron and iron-binding capacity.

5.8   Exogenous factors

As outlined in detail in Chapter 2, there are a great number of preanalytical exogenous factors that affect clinical laboratory test results and many of these influence reference values, including:

food intake	alcohol intake
posture	stress
pregnancy	exercise
immobilization	drug administration
previous medical and surgical care	

5.9   Genetic factors

Certain disease states are more common in different areas in the world and knowledge of particular difficulties that might arise in the population served will be of great value to the individual laboratory. An excellent example is that provided by Walmsley and White (*see* Further reading[8]) regarding the reference values appropriate to Australian aboriginals. Aboriginals often have low levels of thyroxine-binding globulin and the low total thyroxine levels found reflect only this, not the presence of hypothyroidism.

Differences in the levels of body constituents can be shown

to occur in individuals of different racial origin, for example, serum albumin is lower in blacks than whites and serum immunoglobulins and creatinine kinase are higher. This may not be truly due to race since blacks in general have lower nutritional standards and are likelier to be employed in manual labour requiring muscular effort. It may also be that some of these apparent effects are simply environmental in origin. Evidence for this particular hypothesis is that individuals who change country of residence may change their body constituent levels to those found in the indigenous population; examples are that serum cholesterol levels rise in Asians who settle in America and immunoglobulin levels fall in Africans who become domiciled in European countries.

5.10   Generation of reference values

In view of the difficulties with (i) the statistical manipulation of data which do not have a true Gaussian (or log-Gaussian) distribution, (ii) the often implied or desired relationships between reference values, health and disease and (iii) the plethora of factors which affect the results of clinical laboratory tests, the generation of relevant reference values is a most difficult subject for which, at this point in time, there are no clear cut definitive answers.

There are two currently favoured approaches. The first is to select very carefully a small number of people (say 120) who fall within groups which prior study of the literature has shown to be desirable for subclassification (for example, men and women, young and elderly). Individuals who pass strict exclusion criteria can then have specimens collected under carefully controlled conditions, the specimens can be analysed and reference values generated. The second approach is to select a large number of people (say 1000) and collect specimens carefully from all of them. After analysis, the data is examined, the strict exclusion criteria applied, the data subclassified into the appropriate groups as determined from prior examination of the literature and reference values then generated. These approaches have been called the *a priori* and *a posteriori* approaches by Siest (*see* Further reading[4]).

The criteria for exclusion of subjects who cannot be used for production of reference values are very difficult to set. The Scandinavian Society for Clinical Chemistry, through the Committee on Reference Values, have defined very rigid criteria (*see* Further reading[1]) which do serve as a model. The criteria are:

No diagnosis which is likely to affect the results of the test for which reference values are being derived.

No consumption of drugs which should affect the particular test results.

Clinical laboratory test results which are:

no urinary albumin or glucose

erythrocyte sedimentation rate	≤ 50 years	< 15mm/h (men)
		< 22 mm/h (women)
	> 50 years	< 21 mm/h (men)
		< 29 mm/h (women)

haematocrit ≥ 0.36 (men)
             ≥ 0.31 (women)

cholesterol (serum) ≤ 9.1 mmol/l
triglycerides (serum) ≤ 2.4 mmol/l

No hypertension ≤ 40 years ≤ 95/150 mmHg
                 > 40 years ≤ 100/160 mmHg

Not more than ± 20% of the ideal body weight.

If these criteria are rigidly applied, only a very small

number of randomly selected persons will be able to pass the exclusion process. A more pragmatic approach is that these criteria can be relaxed and reference populations selected with the assessment of tests for particular diseases in mind. For example, a reference sample group for creatine kinase could be selected simply by excluding individuals with evidence of heart attack or muscle diseases, those involved in heavy muscular exercise, pregnant women and patients who have had intramuscular injections.

When selection of subjects, specimen collection and laboratory tests have been completed, reference values are obtained from the data by statistical manipulation. As outlined earlier, the use of traditional parametric statistics has deficiencies and, for this reason, the Expert Panel on Theory of Reference Values has suggested (*see* Further reading[3]) that the *nonparametric central 0.95 interfractile interval* be derived. This is a complex way of stating the simple strategy that all the reference values are listed in order and the lowest and highest 2.5% of values are deleted from each end to give a 95% reference interval. This procedure has the advantage that no assumptions are made regarding the distribution characteristics of the numerical data.

5.11   Reporting of results and reference values

There are many ways in which observed values can be related to reference values. The simplest is of course the widely adopted, and some would have essential, objective thoughtful comparison of appropriate reference values provided along with every test result. This comparison should only be done if the reference values are appropriate. If there are different sets of reference values for different groups (men and women, young and elderly, inpatient and outpatient, etc), the correct values may not in fact, be documented on the laboratory report. Certain clinical laboratories adopt an interesting and useful approach. If there are many sets of reference values, the result is flagged in some way to show this, no particular possibly incorrect set of reference values is printed upon the report and the user of the report is advised to consult the appropriate laboratory handbook provided which lists the complete available sets of reference values.

It is certainly not appropriate to use reference values of dubious origin from textbooks, diaries, commercial material and the like in clinical settings.

Many clinical laboratories flag test results that are outside the reference intervals and classify results into three groups (low, usual and high) or into five groups (very low, low, usual, high and very high) or even more. These approaches have limitations in that (i) the reports may be scanned merely briefly to check whether any tests results are flagged and therefore worthy of attention, (ii) an unflagged result within the reference interval, which may be of great value in aiding or making a diagnosis, assessing prognosis or monitoring therapy, may be missed and (iii), as will be discussed in detail in Chapter 6, a value within the reference interval may be unusual for an individual patient depending upon the usual biological variation around the homeostatic setting point of that individual.

There are many other ways of relating observed and re-ference values. These include the following which have been discussed in detail by Dybkaer (*see* Further reading[3]).

The 'Sta-nine' approach where the reference interval is divided into seven segments (2–8) and 1 and 9 are lower and higher than the reference limits respectively. 'Sta-ten', a minor modification, has 0 below the lower reference limit and 9 above the upper reference limit, 1–8 being subclasses of the reference interval.

The observed value can be divided by the mean of the reference interval or by the upper limit of the interval, either as a figure or, multiplied by 100, as a 'centinormalized unit'.

The strategy termed the 'SD unit', 'normal equivalence deviate' or 'SD difference' is calculated as *observed* value-mean/SD. This may also be used after 10 has been added.

The value $\dfrac{\text{observed value-}\frac{1}{2}\text{ upper reference limit,}}{\frac{1}{2}\text{ lower reference limit}}$

termed the 'relative limit', gives a reference interval of -1 to $+1$. This, added to 10 and then multiplied by 10, is termed the 'normal quotient unit' and the reference interval becomes 90–110 units.

The 'clinical unit' is simpler giving a reference interval of 80–120 since it is

$$10\times(10+\frac{\text{observed value-}\frac{1}{2}\text{ upper reference limit)}}{\frac{1}{4}\text{ (upper-lower reference limit)}}$$

These derived values have had little popular appeal and are rarely used in clinical laboratory practice. The Expert Panel has recommended that, along with the observed value, the statistic that gives the best estimate of the unusualness of the value is the *number fraction* of reference individuals who had values below the observed value; this is called the fractile. For example, a serum sodium reported as 134 mmol/l ($P = 0.011$) means that 1.1% of reference individuals have a serum sodium less than 124 mmol/l and the test result is very unusual. A serum AST activity of 65 U/l ($P = 0.994$) means that 99.4% of reference individuals have a serum AST less than 65 U/l and again this value is unusual, unusually high in this case.

5.12   Problems with reference values

Irrespective of the strategy adopted to derive reference values, traditional reference intervals encompass 95% of the population. This means that *1 in 20* individuals who are healthy will have clinical laboratory test results that are *outside* the reference interval; 2.5% of individuals will have test results lower than the lower reference limit and 2.5% will have test results higher than the upper reference limit. Such individuals may be clinically misclassified if observed values are very strictly compared to reference values and the reference limits actually used as clinical decision making limits.

This has particular ramifications when more than one clinical laboratory test is performed, the usual current practice. The percentage change of finding a result outside reference intervals can be calculated from the formula:

$$\text{percentage chance} = (1-0.95^{\text{number of tests}})\times 100$$

which results as shown in Table 5.2.

Table 5.2.

No. of tests	Percentage chance of a result outside reference intervals
1	5
2	10
3	14
4	19
5	23
10	40
20	64

This is, as discussed in Chapter 1, one of the reasons why performing clinical chemistry tests in a profiling mode has disadvantages.

The above calculation does assume that the tests performed are truly independent. This is not the case since many tests are interdependent in some way, for example, sodium and chloride, calcium and phosphate, and urea and creatine. The situation in real clinical practice therefore becomes somewhat less serious and the results shown in Table 5.3 have been calculated:

Table 5.3.

No. of tests	No. of tests with results outside reference intervals
2–7	1
8–16	2
17–28	3
29–40	4
41–52	5

In addition, as will be discussed in detail in Chapter 6, the biological variation of individuals around their own homeostatic setting points means that multiple results from one individual of a single clinical laboratory test may be (i) always within the reference interval, (ii) both within and outside the interval or (iii) always outside the interval.

5.13 Summary

Traditional concepts regarding the use and generation of normal values are suspect and a new terminology has recently been introduced which covers all aspects of reference value theory. The ubiquitous correct use of this terminology would undoubtedly improve the understanding of both this facet of clinical laboratory practice and the interpretation of results.

Many factors affect reference values and these can be classified as analytical, endogenous, exogenous and genetic. The many factors mean that appropriate reference values must always be used in clinical practice and it is the role of the clinical laboratory to provide these. Generation of reference values is complex however and very careful attention must be paid to selection of reference individuals, specimen collection, analytical techniques and data reduction.

Comparison of observed values with reference values can be performed using a variety of both simple and complex mathematical techniques. Consideration of the individual patient by the clinician, along with knowledge of appropriate reference values, will, in most cases, allow correct interpretation.

Further reading

1   Alstrom T., Grasbeck R., Hjelm M. & Skandsen S. (1975) Recommendations concerning the collection of reference values in clinical chemistry and activity report. *Scandinavian Journal of Clinical and Laboratory Investigation,* **35** (Supplement 144), 1.

2   Barnett R.N. (1971) *Clinical Laboratory Statistics.* Little, Brown and Co., Boston.

3   Dybkaer R. (1982) The theory of reference values. Part 6. Presentation of observed values related to reference values. *Journal of Clinical Chemistry and Clinical Biochemistry,* **20,** 841.

4   Grasbeck R. & Alstrom T. Eds. (1981) *Reference Values in Laboratory Medicine. The Current State of the Art.* John Wiley and Sons, Chichester.
    This excellent thought-provoking book describes the papers presented, discussion and outcome of a Workshop held under the auspices of Nordkem in 1980. The material referred to in this chapter written by Grasbeck, Siest and Dybkaer and the data from the Sherbrooke study can be found therein.

5   Grasbeck R., Siest G., Wilding P., Williams G.Z. & Whitehead T.P. (1978) Provisional recommendation on the theory of reference values. Part 1. The concept of

reference values. *Clinica chimica acta,* **87,** 459.

6   Meites S. Ed. (1981) *Pediatric Clinical Chemistry.* 2nd Edition. The American Association for Clinical Chemistry, Washington.

7   Murphy E.A.S (1972) The normal and the perils of the sylleptic argument. *Perspectives in Biology and Medicine,* **15,** 566.

8   Walmsley R.N. & White G.H. (1983) *A Guide to Diagnostic Clinical Chemistry.* Blackwell Scientific Publications Ltd., Melbourne.

Chapter 6

Biological Variation

6.1 Introduction

The results of clinical laboratory tests performed on individuals often do change with time. In disease states, the changes seen may parallel the severity of disease or may give clues to the success or otherwise of treatment or to the likely outcome. It is important that the time scales of these changes be recognized clearly. For example, serum creatine kinase activity will be likely within reference values on the fourth day after myocardial infarction; this test is therefore of little value in aiding in the making of a diagnosis four or more days after the onset of chest pain. On the other hand, because of the rapid fall to usual levels, the test is of considerable value in detection of reinfarction when further chest pain occurs in hospitalized patients with marked electrocardiographic changes. A further example is the change in serum amylase activity that occurs following an episode of acute pancreatitis; for example, a 35-year-old male had the following results, the appropriate reference interval for serum amylase activity being 70–300 U/l;

	Units	On admission	Day 1	Day 2	Day 3	Day 7
Amylase	U/l	3580	14820	6430	1668	297

The results fall, as is usual, to within reference limits on days 3–6. This test is therefore not useful in the assessment of abdominal pain which occurred some days prior to hopsitalization, but the fall to within reference limits by day 7 provides some evidence that there is no serious coexisting abdominal pathology.

Knowledge of these temporal changes with disease is vital to the appropriate clinical selection of laboratory tests and to the correct interpretation of results. Such changes are dealt with in those texts describing clinical aspects of the use of clinical biochemistry tests and do not fall within the scope of this text.

Many predictable changes in results with time occur after physiological or pharmacological stimulation or suppression. These changes are made use of in clinical laboratory practice and are the basis of dynamic function testing. This type of test, although not usually routinely performed, has many advantages. The response of an individual is being compared to the basal level in that individual in addition to being interpreted in relation to results found in both reference individuals and diseased persons. A good knowledge of the usual changes in results with time is required for correct interpretation. For example, in a synacthen test in an 86-year-old male treated with long-term steroid therapy for asthma, the results were

	0900	0930	1000	1030	Units
serum cortisol	230	361	528	557	nmol/l

Usually, results at 0900 hr would fall within the reference interval of 270–625 nmol/l and the concentration would rise to a peak value at 30–60 minutes after stimulation by synacthen and then fall. The interpretation of the results requires knowledge of this time scale because the low first result and the *delayed* response show that, although the patient had impairment of cortisol production, the ability to respond adequately to exogenous adrenocorticotrophin (ACTH) was still present, an important finding from the clinical point of view.

Further interesting examples can be found again in texts dealing with diagnostic clinical laboratory tests.

6.2   Biological rhythms

Changes in the levels of body constituents do occur with time in situations other than in disease and following stimulation or suppression. As discussed in detail in Chapter 5, changes in the results of laboratory tests occur in individuals as they age, particularly important periods being the neonatal period, childhood and old age. Other more regular rhythmic changes occur and these may be of a daily, monthly or seasonal nature.

Daily rhythms

Many serum and urine constituents show changes during the day. These daily rhythms may be classified as diurnal, where the variation occurs depending on the time of day, or nychthemeral, where the variation is dependent on the sleep–wake cycle. Certain of these changes are regular and these include those seen in serum cortisol, growth hormone and prolactin levels as shown in Fig. 6.1. The changes during the day are not really as smooth as those shown in this figure (and in similar diagrams in other texts) because secretion of hormone does occur in an episodic manner during the entire 24 hour period in addition to the general biological rhythmic changes. An example is shown in Fig. 6.2 which displays the mean and 95% tolerance interval of serum TSH concentration in seven individuals who were healthy and euthyroid and demonstrates the episodic secretion superimposed on the daily rhythm.

It is important to note that the peaks and troughs seen during the day do not occur at the same times for all hormones, cortisol peaking at the time of waking, growth hormone reaching a maximum soon after sleeping begins, prolactin rising slowly during sleep and falling during the two hours after waking and TSH reaching maximum concen-

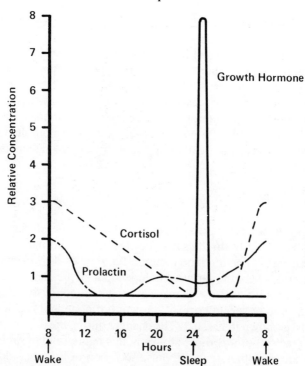

Fig. 6.1. Average smoothed changes in serum cortisol, growth hormone and prolactin levels during a typical 24 hour period demonstrating a variety of daily rhythms.

trations during the first half of the sleep period.

These daily rhythms may not be regular throughout life. Very high growth hormone concentrations are present in the first few days of life, peaks of high growth hormone levels occur during the day and after exercise in the pubertal period and the sleep peak may be reduced or absent in the elderly, for example.

Other hormones, including serum testosterone in men, serum renin and aldosterone and urinary 17-oxo- and oxo-

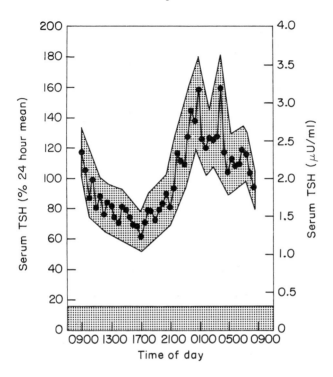

Fig. 6.2. Daily rhythm of serum TSH in healthy euthyroid subjects. Blood was drawn at half-hourly intervals and assayed for TSH. The mean TSH concentration is expressed both as the absolute concentration (right hand scale) and as a percentage of the average 24 hour TSH concentration (left hand scale). Each point is the mean of the values of 7 subjects for that time. The shaded area about the points represents the 95% tolerance for the mean. The shaded area at the bottom indicates the minimal detectable serum concentration. From Wehmann R.E. and Nisula B.C. (1984) *CRC Critical Reviews in Clinical Laboratory Sciences*, **20**, 257 (with permission).

genic steroids also show marked cyclical rhythms of a daily nature.

Similar apparently daily rhythms may be due to exogenous factors. The changes related to posture documented in detail in Chapter 2 also happen when sleep occurs. Further minor daily changes in body constituents are well documented by Young (*see* Further reading[7]).

Knowledge of these rhythms is important in (i) the collection of specimens, because reference values are well documented only at certain times of day and since observed values are very often compared with reference values by both clinicians and laboratories (*see* Chapter 5), it is essential to collect specimens at these times and (ii) the detection and monitoring of disease, because the rhythms may be altered or abolished in such circumstances. As examples, the daily rhythm of TSH is absent in severe hypothyroidism, the sleep peak of growth hormone is absent in both acromegaly and deficiency states and the expected rhythm of cortisol may be absent in Cushing's syndrome. The serum cortisol level at midnight is usually less than 270 nmol/l or is less than ½ the level at 0900 hr. A 61-year-old male had the following results:

serum cortisol: 0900	683 nmol/l
serum cortisol: 2400	419 nmol/l

On further investigation (which included assay or urinary cortisol: 941 nmol/day—reference interval—up to 600 nmol/day), the hypersecretion of cortisol was found to be due to excess pituitary secretion of ACTH.

Although taking a *single* specimen for investigation of the level of a constituent that has a marked biological rhythm will have to be very much constrained by time considerations, many dynamic function tests can be performed at a convenient time of day because the numerical change, on stimulation or suppression, is essentially unaffected by time. For example, three synacthen tests were performed on a patient in the morning, afternoon and evening; the serum cortisol results are shown in Table 6.1.

Table 6.1.

	Morning	Afternoon	Evening
Cortisol before test	529 nmol/l	364 nmol/l	224 nmol/l
Cortisol after test	938 nmol/l	840 nmol/l	686 nmol/l
Increment	409 nmol/l	476 nmol/l	462 nmol/l

As expected, the basal serum cortisol levels fall during the day but the incremental rise is consistent no matter when the test is performed.

Monthly rhythms

The most important monthly cycles are those found in women during the reproductive phase of life. Examples are the changes in serum levels of luteotrophin (luteinizing hormone, LH), oestradiol and progesterone, which are shown in Fig. 6.3. Many other hormonal changes are also found and these, and other changes, have again been documented in detail by Young (*see* Further reading[7]). As with daily rhythms, it is essential to be cogniscent of these monthly rhythms so that specimens can be collected at the time most appropriate for the purpose of the particular clinical investigation and appropriate reference intervals can be provided and used. Changes from the expected rhythms can also be of considerable value in the investigation of disease and in assessment of the success of treatment of fertility problems, although many investigations of hormonal status are best dealt with by dynamic function tests.

Seasonal rhythms

Although most of the changes seen during the menstrual cycle

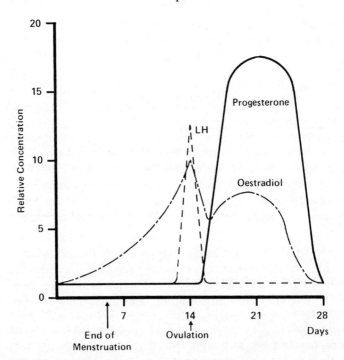

Fig. 6.3. Average smoothed changes in serum LH, oestradiol and progesterone levels during a typical 28 day menstrual cycle.

are hormonal in nature, many of the changes seen during the day in constituents which are not hormones can be attributed to exogenous factors such as posture, meals and times of sleeping and waking. Similarly, most of the seasonal rhythms are probably due to exogenous factors. Examples are the increase in the summer found in serum lactate dehydrogenase activity and urinary adrenal hormone metabolites which are probably due to exercise, the increase in serum cholesterol levels during the winter which is possibly due to dietary effects and the increased plasma volume in summer which is likely due to the increased ambient temperature of the environment causing significant vasodilatation. Probably the seasonal variations best documented are the marked changes in the vitamin D metabolite, serum 25-hydroxycholecalciferol, where levels are higher in summer (particularly in countries far from the equator); this is related to the weather but UV-B radiation rather than sunshine is probably the best indicator. Thus, in addition to a cyclical variation in serum levels, there is year to year variation due to the yearly differences in the levels of UV-B radiation and this is shown for two years in Fig. 6.4.

As with daily and monthly rhythms, the interpretation of clinical laboratory test results cannot be performed correctly without taking biological variations of a cyclical nature into account.

6.3 Random biological variation

In contrast to those body constituents which show rhythmic daily, monthly, or seasonal variation, most of interest to the clinician and the laboratory do not show cyclical changes. Although a number of mathematical models have been proposed to describe the variation of such constituents, particularly by Harris (*see* Further reading[3]), the simplest model is to consider that the variation is random and can thus be described using parametric (Gaussian) statistics.

If the serum sodium was measured on six days in a young adult male, typical results would be:

Units	Day 1	Day 2	Day 3	Day 4	Day 5	Day 6
mmol/l	138	137	139	140	137	141

The variation seen in the numerical results is due to two sources of variation: analytical imprecision (*see* Chapter 4) and biological variation of a random nature. This biological variation is due to both the intrinsic homeostatic variation around

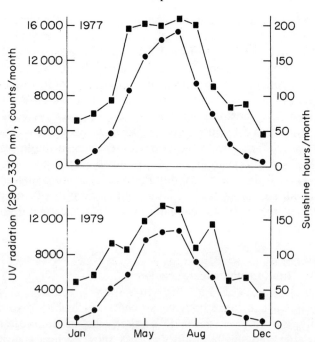

Fig. 6.4. Relationship between sunshine hours (■) and ultraviolet radiation in the range 290–330 nm (●) between the months of January and December as measured in Dundee (latitude 56° 36′ N). The coefficient of correlation between sunshine hours and UV–B radiation was 0.96 for 1977 and 0.94 for 1979. From Devgun M.S. *et al.* (1983) *Clinical Physiology and Biochemistry*, **1**, 303 (with permission).

the biological *setting-point* and to the many preanalytical factors and sample collection factors such as posture, previous intake of food and drink, exercise, tourniquet application time and the like (*see* Chapters 2 and 3).

A second individual is similarly examined for six days and

the results of serum sodium analyses are:

Units	Day 1	Day 2	Day 3	Day 4	Day 5	Day 6
mmol/l	142	140	143	141	142	144

Again the variation arises from analytical and biological sources.

It can be seen by visual inspection that both individuals vary but that they have different inherent levels of serum sodium. This is described using the following terminology: the biological variation around the homeostatic setting-point is called the *intraindividual biological variation* and the difference between the setting-points of individuals is called the *interindividual biological variation*.

6.4 Determination of components and variation

Biological variation data have a number of valuable applications. The data can be determined by careful attention to both experimental design and execution and to statistical analysis.

In a typical study, a small but statistically valid group of individuals is selected. To determine biological variation in the healthy, it is usual to attempt to minimize some of the factors influencing clinical laboratory test results by ensuring that overt disease is not present, no drugs that might affect the test results are being taken and a usual life-style is being followed. In addition, the preparation of the subjects prior to specimen collection is carefully controlled and the collection itself is performed under standardized conditions in order to minimize sources of preanalytical variation.

A series of specimens is taken from each subject and the specimen handling procedures kept constant throughout. After processing, the specimens are stored in a manner which ensures stability.

Analysis is performed following a rigid protocol. Each set of specimens from an individual subject is analysed in a single batch preferably with a single lot number of reagents and consumables being used by a single operator using one instrument or analytical technique. Each set is then randomized and reanalysed.

From the duplicate analyses, the analytical imprecision (SD_A) can be calculated using the formula:

$$SD_A = \sqrt{\frac{\text{sum of (differences)}^2}{2 \times \text{no. of pairs}}}$$

For each individual, a *single* set of data is used to calculate the SD, which is made up of analytical and intraindividual biological variation (SD_I),

$$SD^2 = SD_A{}^2 + SD_I{}^2$$

the squared SD (variance) being used because variance is the statistic which can be mathematically manipulated. The average intraindividual biological variation can then be calculated.

From the SD for all single sets of data of all subjects, which is comprised of analytical, intraindividual and interindividual biological variation (SD_G),

$$SD^2 = SD_A{}^2 + SD_I{}^2 + SD_G{}^2$$

the interindividual variation can be calculated. The approach is shown diagramatically in Fig. 6.5.

6.5 Magnitude of biological variation

A number of well designed and executed studies have documented the biological variation of serum constituents in the healthy. The data have been summarized by Ross (*see* Further reading[5]). The consensus intra- and interindividual variations

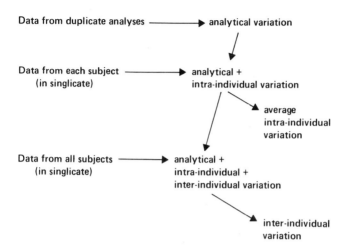

Fig. 6.5. Strategy used to determine components of biological variation.

as coefficients of variation (CV) are shown in Table 6.2; these are the values found over a 2–22 week time span and are the means of the literature values tabulated. There is a paucity of data in the literature on endocrinological clinical laboratory tests and only one study on the components of biological variation of urinary constituents; short (2 days), medium (5 days) and longer (5 months) term variations of ten urinary constituents are shown (in SD terms) in Table 6.3; the data are from Shephard *et al.* (*see* Further reading[6]).

6.6 Biological variation in hospitalized patients

There are less data available concerning the components of biological variation in hospitalized patients than are available from healthy individuals and yet most test results are obtained on the former group. However, studies have been performed

Table 6.2. Average intra- and interindividual biological variation of some serum constituents in healthy individuals over 2 to 22 weeks; data taken from literature sources and expressed as CV.

Serum constituent	Intraindividual variation	Interindividual variation
Sodium	0.7	0.6
Potassium	5.1	4.4
Calcium	1.7	2.2
Magnesium	2.2	5.9
Chloride	1.7	1.4
Bicarbonate	4.6	3.0
Urea	13.6	16.9
Creatinine	4.6	10.6
Urate	8.6	13.4
Phosphate	7.8	9.4
Bilirubins	25.1	35.2
Iron	26.8	23.5
Cholesterol	5.5	14.8
Triglycerides	27.3	52.2
Glucose	6.2	6.4
Proteins	2.7	3.7
Albumin	3.1	3.3
Acid phosphatase	8.9	8.0
Alkaline phosphatase	6.7	25.4
Alanine aminotransferase	39.4	52.7
Aspartate aminotransferase	16.3	20.4
Creatine kinase	71.6	67.7
Gamma-glutamyltransferase	34.7	86.7
Lactate dehydrogenase	7.6	14.7
Total thyroxine	10.1	18.0

on patients with myocardial infarction, renal failure, pregnant women with a variety of diseases, multiple sclerosis and pyelonephritis. These have shown fortunately that the intra-individual biological variation of serum constituents in the ill is of the same order as in the healthy. This applies irrespective

Table 6.3. Average intraindividual biological variation of urinary constituents in apparently healthy young men over short (2 days), medium (5 days) and longer (5 months) terms, expressed as SD.

Constituent	Units	Short term	Medium term	Longer term
Sodium	mmol/l	49.7	35.3	29.3
Potassium	mmol/l	30.7	19.8	15.4
Osmolality	mmol/kg	139.8	132.3	137.2
Urea	mmol/l	80.9	71.7	91.2
Creatinine	mmol/l	5.6	3.5	3.8
Calcium	mmol/l	2.0	1.2	1.3
Phosphate	mmol/l	14.7	6.5	8.7
Proteins	g/l	0.02	0.02	0.02
Glucose	mmol/l	0.2	0.1	0.1
Urate	mmol/l	1.4	1.1	0.9

of whether the levels are within the appropriate reference limits (for example, serum sodium in patients with myocardial infarction), outside such limits (for example, serum creatinine in patients with impairment of renal function) or affected by usual physiological changes (for example, serum urea and albumin in pregnant women). This is perhaps not unexpected since, except in acute clinical situations, the variation around the biological setting-point may be considered unlikely to alter although the setting-point itself may change.

The practical ramification of these conclusions is that the data available on biological variation in the healthy can be applied validly in the various clinical uses of such data.

6.7 Uses of biological variation data

Biological variation data can be used (i) to assess the significance of changes in serial tests results obtained on an individual patient, (ii) determine the usefulness or otherwise of conventional population based reference values and (iii) delineate the minimum acceptable performance standards required for clinical laboratory analyses.

Significance of changes

As alluded to in Chapter 4, the probability that two test results from a single patient are statistically significantly different can be based upon the SD (imprecision) of the test (Table 6.4).

Table 6.4.

Difference between results	Probability that results differ
1.5 SD	$< 70\%$
2.0 SD	$< 90\%$
2.5 SD	$< 95\%$
2.8 SD	$= 95\%$
3.0 SD	$> 95\%$
3.5 SD	$> 98\%$
4.0 SD	$> 99\%$

However, in reality, the difference between two results from an individual patient is not only due to analytical random variation but also biological variation. The total variation required for a significant change to have occurred can be calculated by addition of the variances, as discussed previously,

$$SD = \sqrt{SD^2_{analytical} + SD^2_{biological,}}$$

and, to be 95% certain that two results are different, this SD must be multiplied by 2.8.

The differences required for some commonly analysed serum constituents are shown in Table 6.5 using the imprecision of the average United Kingdom laboratory (Table

4.1) and the average intraindividual biological variation (Table 6.2). The differences are documented for the levels shown, which are approximately the mid-points of reference intervals quoted in the United Kingdom.

Table 6.5. The change required for serum constituents in two specimens from an individual to differ significantly.

Serum constituent	Level	Units	Change required
Sodium	140	mmol/l	6
Potassium	4.2	mmol/l	0.6
Calcium	2.40	mmol/l	0.19
Magnesium	1.0	mmol/l	0.4
Chloride	100	mmol/l	6
Bicarbonate	26	mmol/l	4
Urea	5.0	mmol/l	2.1
Creatinine	60	μmol/l	21
Urate	0.26	mmol/l	0.07
Phosphate	1.2	mmol/l	0.3
Bilirubins	10	μmol/l	10
Iron	18	μmol/l	8
Cholesterol	5.8	mmol/l	1.6
Triglycerides	1.2	mmol/l	0.9
Glucose	4.6	mmol/l	1.6
Proteins	75	g/l	6
Albumin	40	g/l	5
Alkaline phosphatase	60	U/l	22
Aspartate aminotransferase	20	U/l	13
Lactate dehydrogenase	125	U/l	57

The differences required for a significant change to have occurred in urinary constituents, calculated from the average imprecision of Australasian laboratories achieved in 1983 (Table 4.2) and the medium term intraindividual biological variation are shown in Table 6.6.

As an example of the use of the data, two serum specimens taken on consecutive days from a 58-year-old man showed the test results in Table 6.7; the differences are also shown. The differences marked by an asterix are statistically significant ($P \geq 0.5$); the differences not so high-lighted, although numerically not the same, are not significant. This is a most important point in the interpretation of clinical laboratory test results. Just because the numerical values have changed does not necessarily mean that the patient is improving or deteriorating or that the therapeutic regime is effective.

Table 6.6. The change required for urinary constituents in two specimens from an individual to differ significantly.

Urinary constituent	Units	Change required
Sodium	mmol/l	99
Potassium	mmol/l	56
Osmolality	mmol/kg	375
Urea	mmol/l	204
Creatinine	mmol/l	10
Calcium	mmol/l	3.4
Phosphate	mmol/l	18
Proteins	g/l	0.3
Glucose	mmol/l	2.3
Urate	mmol/l	3.4

For serum constituents, the data here will generally be valid for clinical use since the imprecision data were derived from analyses of materials which had levels which did include those used for calculation in Table 6.2. In contrast, the urinary data are given for completeness but are less valid. The biological variation data are from one study only. The imprecision data were derived from analyses of materials which had values covering a very wide range of levels.

Table 6.7.

Constituent	Units	Day 1	Day 2	Difference	
Sodium	mmol/l	140	144	4	
Potassium	mmol/l	4.2	4.9	0.7	*
Chloride	mmol/l	101	103	2	
Bicarbonate	mmol/l	24	29	5	*
Urea	mmol/l	6.2	6.8	0.6	
Creatinine	μmol/l	105	115	10	
Calcium	mmol/l	2.25	2.47	0.23*	
Phosphate	mmol/l	1.1	1.4	0.3	
Proteins	g/l	74	81	7	*
Albumin	g/l	38	44	6	*
Alkaline phosphatase	U/l	82	106	24	*

Moreover, the data presented here for serum and urinary constituents do assume that the laboratory achieves the average analytical performance. It is therefore important for individual clinical laboratories to thoroughly document the imprecisions achieved in their own laboratory and to provide this information to the users of test results so that better interpretation of numerical data can be achieved with good knowledge of both relevant analytical and biological variation. Furthermore, it must be remembered that the data, particularly those in Table 6.2, are average data and, as will be discussed in the next section of this chapter, individuals do have very different intraindividual biological variation for certain constituents.

Reference values

The availability of data on intra- and interindividual biological variation has allowed objective assessment of the value of population based reference values.

Weekly measurements of serum potassium in 37 healthy men over a 22 week period were performed by Pickup and associates (*see* Further reading[4]). The results were displayed as shown in Fig. 6.6. Each horizontal bar represents the range of results for each individual and the circle depicts the mean. The vertical dashed lines denote the reference limits calculated from all of the data. It can be seen that the means for all individuals fall within the reference interval and the intra-individual biological variation of the subjects is generally of the same order. It is important to note that, while most results do fall within the reference interval, some do not. Healthy individuals can and do have test results which lie outside the reference interval and this simple (but often unappreciated) fact must be remembered when results are interpreted and used for clinical purposes.

The same data are shown for alkaline phosphatase activity in Fig. 6.7. It can be seen, in marked contrast to serum potassium, that different individuals have markedly different mean values, the variations around the means are sometimes large and sometimes small and certain individuals do have results outside the conventional reference interval. For constituents which have this type of pattern, reference values will not be of significant help to interpretation because individuals may have marked changes with constituent levels significantly different from their own usual values but all these results may still lie within the usual reference interval. Thus, if intra-individual biological variation is greater than interindividual variation, conventional population based reference values will (with many caveats) be of value. However, if inter-individual biological variation is greater than intraindividual variation, then such reference values will be of limited use and may, indeed, give misleading impressions.

This concept has been more formally stated by Harris (*see*

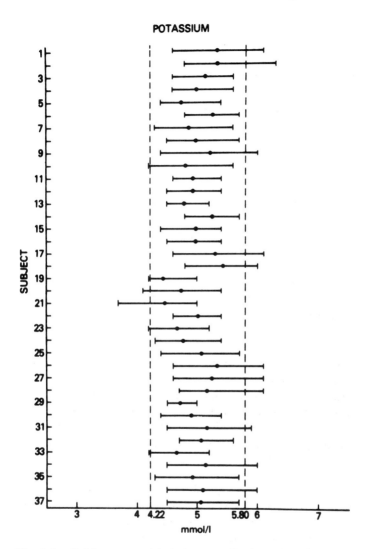

Fig. 6.6. Subject means (circles), ranges (horizontal bars) and reference limits (dotted lines) for serum potassium in 37 healthy subjects. From Pickup J.F. *et al.* (1977) *Clinical Chemistry,* **23,** 842 (with permission).

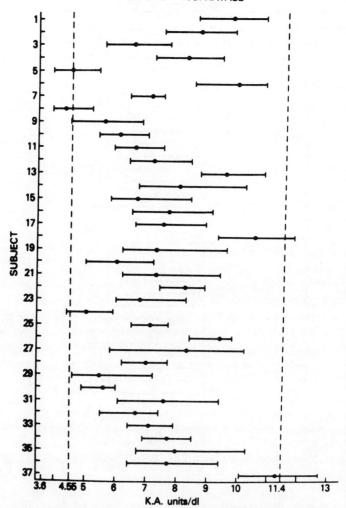

Fig. 6.7. Subject means (circles), ranges (horizontal bars) and reference limits (dotted lines) for serum alkaline phosphatase in 37 healthy subjects. From Pickup J.F. *et al.* (1977) *Clinical Chemistry,* **23,** 842 (with permission).

Further reading[2]). A ratio can be calculated from:

$$\sqrt{\frac{(\mathrm{SD}_{\mathrm{intraindividual}})^2}{(\mathrm{SD}_{\mathrm{interindividual}})^2}}$$

When this ratio is high, particularly when greater than 1.4, conventional reference values are of most use. When the ratio is low, particularly when less than 0.6, conventional reference values are of little relevance to correct interpretation of results; comparison of test results with those obtained previously on the same individual would be of greater value.

The ratios can be calculated from the data shown in Table 6.2. Serum magnesium, creatinine, cholesterol, triglycerides, alkaline phosphatase, gamma-glutamyltransferase, lactate dehydrogenase, thyroxine and other indices of thyrometabolic status have low ratios and are said to have a high degree of individuality. Serum sodium, potassium, chloride and bicarbonate have low degrees of individuality.

For urinary constituents, urea and osmolality show high individuality but sodium, urate, phosphate and glucose exhibit low degrees of individuality.

Laboratory performance standards

Although the setting of *analytical goals* for the performance characteristics of tests (that is the minimum acceptable standards to provide good patient care) is somewhat controversial, it is accepted by most interested in this aspect of clinical laboratory work that goals for imprecision should be based upon biological variation. This is based upon the premise that analytical imprecision should not widen unduly reference intervals and should also allow real changes in individual patients to be more easily monitored. If biological variation around the homeostatic setting-point is small, low analytical imprecision will be required.

For short-term imprecision and for monitoring individuals, mathematically, the goal is expressed as:

$$SD_{analytical} \leq \tfrac{1}{2}SD_{intraindividual}$$

This topic is mainly of interest to the clinical laboratory and to clinicians responsible for performing tests. It will therefore not be dealt with in more detail here. A full up-to-date exposition can be found in the article by Fraser (*See* Further reading[1]).

6.8 Summary

Changes in numerical laboratory results can occur in a predictable manner with time following acute disease processes. Further predictable changes in test results follow physiological or pharmacological stimulation or suppression. Changes also occur over a lifetime and are particularly marked during the neonatal period and childhood and in the elderly. Certain constituents have rhythmical variation which may be daily, monthly or seasonal in nature.

Knowledge of these changes is vital so that specimens may be collected at appropriate times, relevant reference values used and correct interpretation of test results facilitated. In addition, the absence of expected temporal changes may provide useful diagnostic or monitoring information.

Most analytes do not exhibit rhythmical variation but rather, in the simplest model at least, show random variation around homeostatic setting-points. The variation around the setting-point is termed the intraindividual variation and the difference between the setting-points is termed the interindividual variation. Data on biological variation is available for many constituents and can be validly used in patient care to assess the significance of serial results obtained on an individual, to determine the usefulness or otherwise of conventional population based reference values and to set desirable standards of analytical performance.

Further reading

1 Fraser C.G. (1983) Desirable performance standards for clinical chemistry tests. *Advances in Clinical Chemistry*, **23,** 299.
2 Harris E.K. (1974) Effects of intra- and interindividual variation on the appropriate use of normal ranges. *Clinical Chemistry*, **20,** 1535.
3 Harris E.K. (1976) Some theory of reference values. II. Comparison of some statistical models of intraindividual variation in blood constituents. *Clinical Chemistry*, **22,** 1343.
4 Pickup J.F., Harris E.K., Kearns M. & Brown S.S. (1977) Intraindividual variation of some serum constituents and its relevance to population-based reference ranges. *Clinical Chemistry*, **23,** 842.
5 Ross J.W. (1982) Evaluation of precision. In Werner M. Ed. *CRC Handbook of Clinical Chemistry. Volume 1.* pp. 391–422. CRC Press, Boca Raton.
6 Shephard M.D.S., Penberthy L.A. & Fraser C.G. (1981) Short- and long-term biological variation in analytes in urine of apparently healthy individuals. *Clinical Chemistry*, **27,** 1939.
7 Young D.S. (1979) Biological variability. In Brown S.S., Mitchell F.L. & Young D.S. Eds. *Chemical Diagnosis of Disease*, pp. 1–113. Elsevier, Amsterdam.

Chapter 7

The Predictive Value
of Tests

7.1 Introduction

The intrinsic biological variation of individuals and the multiplicity of factors that affect reference values, as discussed in earlier chapters, make the comparison of test results with reference values more difficult than is usually imagined. In addition, the various uses made of the term 'normal' undoubtedly hinder the logical use of test results.

For these reasons, Galen and Gambino applied the *predictive value model* used in epidemiology to clinical laboratory tests and their text, published in 1975 (*see* Further reading[1]), did a great deal to stimulate interest in the objective assessment of the use of laboratory data.

7.2 Definitions

In order to understand and make full use of the predictive value model, an understanding of a number of terms must be gained.

Prevalence is the number of persons who have a particular disease in a particular population.

Incidence is the number of persons who develop a particular disease over a stated period of time.

Sensitivity is the number of results which are true positive results, that is, positive results found in diseased persons. (False positive results are such results found in healthy non-diseased persons).

Specificity is the number of results which are true negative

136

results, that is, negative results found in healthy persons. (False negative results are such results found in diseased persons).

Predictive Value of a positive test is the percentage of all positive results which are true positive results when the test is used for a group of persons which contains both diseased and healthy persons. Similarly, the predictive value of a negative test is the percentage of all negative results which are true negative results.

Efficiency is the percentage of all results that are true results, whether true positive results or true negative results.

7.3 Data analysis

Making use of the predictive value model is straightforward when data on diseased and healthy persons are available. Firstly, the population is divided into four groups:

(i) persons with disease and positive test results—true positives (TP).

(ii) persons with disease but negative test results—false negatives (FN).

(iii) persons without disease but positive test results—false positives (FP).

(iv) persons without disease and negative test results—true negatives (TN).

The four groups are then displayed in a table and both the horizontal and vertical rows totalled (Table 7.1).

Returning to the definitions given above, it is simple to calculate the characteristics of the test, since:

Prevalence = no of persons with disease in the group

$$= \frac{\text{(i)}+\text{(ii)}}{\text{(i)}+\text{(ii)}+\text{(iii)}+\text{(iv)}} = \frac{TP+FN}{TP+FN+FP+TN}$$

Table 7.1.

Disease	Test results		
	Positive	*Negative*	*Totals*
Present	(i) TP	(ii) FN	(i)+(ii) TP+FN
Absent	(iii) FP	(iv) TN	(iii)+(iv) FP+TN
Totals	(i)+(iii) TP+FP	(ii)+(iv) FN+TN	(i)+(ii)+(iii)+(iv) TP+FN+FP+TN

Sensitivity = number of true positive results in the diseased

$$= \frac{(i)}{(i)+(ii)} = \frac{TP}{TP+FN}$$

Specificity = number of true negative results in the healthy

$$= \frac{(iv)}{(iii)+(iv)} = \frac{TN}{FP+TN}$$

Predictive value of a positive test = number of positive test results which are true positives

$$= \frac{(i)}{(i)+(iii)} = \frac{TP}{TP+FP}$$

Predictive value of a negative test = number of negative tests which are true negatives

$$= \frac{(iv)}{(ii)+(iv)} = \frac{TN}{FN+TN}$$

Efficiency = number of true positive and true negative results

$$= \frac{(i)+(iv)}{(i)+(ii)+(iii)+(iv)} = \frac{TP+TN}{TP+FN+FP+TN}$$

All of these characteristics are usually expressed as percentages.

The use of the table can be perhaps more easily remembered using the guide shown in Fig. 7.1.

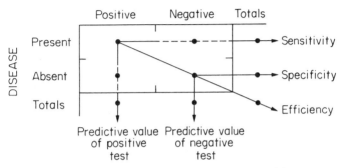

Fig. 7.1. Diagram to aid calculation of predictive model test characteristics. The numerical data from the origin of the arrow is divided by the numerical data outside the rectangular box to give the characteristic at the end of the arrow. Data bracketed by broken lines is not relevant to the particular calculation, but data with solid lines is used.

7.4 Application of the model

Assays of serum or plasma enzyme activities are widely used in the assessment of myocardial infarction. Aspartate aminotransferase activity (AST) is often used because (i) the assay is not complex, (ii) the assay can be easily mechanized, (iii) the reagents are relatively inexpensive and (iv) because AST is widely distributed in the body, the same assay can be used in assessment of other diseases, for example liver disease, which do not cause clinical confusion with myocardial infarction.

In this hypothetical but realistic example, all patients admitted to a coronary care unit over a period of one year have AST assayed on admission to the unit. The data is collected and, using strict criteria (clinical assessment, e.c.g. studies and results of enzyme activity assays *other than AST*) the patients are divided into those who have suffered a myocardial infarction and those who have not. The data can be stratified into groups according to the enzyme activity (Table 7.2).

Table 7.2.

AST Enzyme Activity (U/l)	Number with infarction	Number without infarction
< 15	16	57
16–25	24	23
26–35	35	20
36–45	41	22
45–55	114	18
> 56	620	10
Total	850	150

The upper reference limit quoted by the laboratory is 35 U/l. The data can then be displayed in the tabular format previously described (Table 7.3).

Table 7.3.

	AST enzyme activity		
	> 35 U/l	≤ 35 U/l	*Totals*
Infarction present	775	75	850
Infarction absent	50	100	150
Totals	825	175	1000

The characteristics of the test can then be calculated.
Prevalence = number of persons with myocardial infarction in the population studied

$$= \frac{850}{1000} \times 100 = 85\%$$

Sensitivity = number of true positive results in the diseased

$$= \frac{775}{850} \times 100 = 91\%$$

Specificity = number of true negative results in the healthy

$$= \frac{100}{150} \times 100 = 67\%$$

Predictive value of a positive test = number of positive results which are true positives

$$= \frac{775}{825} \times 100 = 94\%$$

Predictive value of a negative test = number of negative results which are true negatives

$$= \frac{100}{175} \times 100 = 57\%$$

Efficiency = numbers of true positives and negatives

$$= \frac{875}{1000} \times 100 = 88\%$$

It is evident that AST, in this particular situation, is good at picking up cases of myocardial infarction (high sensitivity) but there are both false positive and false negative results. Indeed, one third of the patients without myocardial infarction would be misclassified as diseased if AST was the criterion of disease since the specificity is 67%.

At this point, it is necessary to consider the definition of disease since the predictive value model, being concerned with the assessment of the clinical value of laboratory tests, depends upon being able to classify persons very clearly as being diseased or healthy. This may be very difficult and the test under study may in fact be a better indicator of disease than any other criteria used. This subject has been recently discussed in detail in an excellent article by Zweig and Robertson (*see* Further reading[5]). Other important aspects include (i) the simple but often overlooked point that the classification of the presence or absence of disease must not be based upon the clinical laboratory test being studied, (ii) in comparisons of different tests, the same subjects and the same specimens should be used, (iii) appropriate patients must be selected for any study and (iv) strictly, the reference limits chosen when comparing clinical laboratory tests should be selected to give the same sensitivity if specificity is being examined and vice versa. It is particularly crucial to remember these considerations when assessing the value and conclusions of publications dealing with the utility of clinical laboratory tests.

7.5 Sensitivity and specificity

Inspection of the data on AST shows that, by selecting the usual population-based upper reference limit, cases of myocardial infarction are missed, some patients with the disease having an AST less than 35 U/l. Moreover, some individuals who have not suffered a myocardial infarction do have AST more than 35 U/l. The question then arises, does alteration of the reference limit improve the test? In order to classify correctly a higher proportion of patients with myocardial infarction, it will be necessary to lower the upper reference limit.

If the upper reference limit was 25 U/l, then the table

becomes as shown in Table 7.4.

Table 7.4.

	AST enzyme activity		
	> 25 U/l	*≤ 25 U/l*	*Totals*
Infarction present	810	40	850
Infarction absent	70	80	150
Totals	*880*	*120*	*1000*

The characteristics of the test are then:

Prevalence $= \dfrac{850}{1000} \times 100 = 85\%$ (unchanged)

Sensitivity $= \dfrac{810}{850} \times 100 = 95\%$ (increased)

Specificity $= \dfrac{80}{150} \times 100 = 53\%$ (decreased)

Predictive value of a positive test $= \dfrac{810}{880} \times 100 = 92\%$ (decreased)

Predictive value of a negative test $= \dfrac{80}{120} \times 100 = 67\%$ (increased)

Efficiency $= \dfrac{890}{1000} \times 100 = 89\%$ (increased)

Alteration of the upper reference does improve the sensitivity of the test, more patients who do have myocardial infarction having a positive test. Unfortunately, adoption of this strategy means that, since there is overlap between test results found in diseased and healthy persons, inevitably the specificity deteriorates, more of the healthy being misclassified as diseased.

This highlights the very important point that *sensitivity and specificity are inversely related.* This is shown in Fig. 7.2. The upper diagram shows a test with high sensitivity; this means that the test classifies most diseased persons correctly (many true positive results and few false negative results). Since sensitivity and specificity have this inverse relationship, such a test will classify healthy people incorrectly as diseased, that is, the specificity will be low with a high number of false positive results. The lower diagram shows the converse situation, that is, a test with low sensitivity (few true positive results and many false negative results) and high specificity (few false positives).

It is important to note that the characteristics derived using the predictive value model can be very much altered by the setting of the upper (or lower) reference limit. Much of the literature which quotes these characteristics does not discuss the influence of the chosen limit and the user of the published data may well have to perform the additional calculations required to make optimal personal use of the experimental results given.

7.6 Predictive value and prevalence

AST assay has high sensitivity and might therefore be considered to be a useful indicator of myocardial infarction. The influence of prevalence of disease on the predictive value of a positive test can be examined by extension of this example; the application of the test to all patients admitted to the hospital is now examined.

As shown previously, in one year, 1000 persons were admitted to the coronary care unit and 850 of these had suffered a myocardial infarction. During the year, a total of 60000 persons are admitted to hospital and all are tested as part of a laboratory admission profile (*see* Chapter 1). It is found that 4000 patients have an AST test result which is

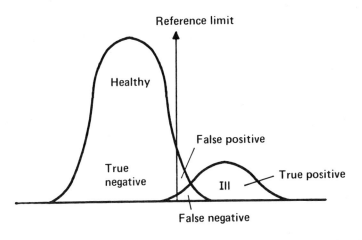

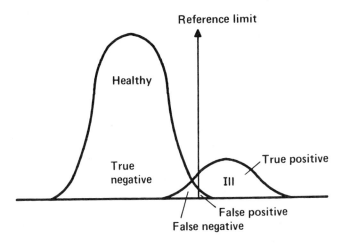

Fig. 7.2. The characteristics of tests with high sensitivity (upper diagram) and high specificity (lower diagram) demonstrating the influence of the reference limit on clinical laboratory test results.

greater than 35 U/l but, on further detailed examination, only 150 of the persons not admitted to the coronary care unit are shown to have had a myocardial infarction. Thus, 1000 persons have actually had an infarction during the year.

The table used to assess the test characteristics can be partly completed with this data (Table 7.5[a]).

Table 7.5 (a).

	AST enzyme activity		
	> 35 U/l	*≤ 35 U/l*	*Totals*
Infarction present	925 (775+150)	75	1000
Infarction absent	—	—	—
Totals	4000	—	60000

The table can then be completed by simple arithmetic (Table 7.5[b]).

Table 7.5(b).

	AST enzyme activity		
	> 35 U/l	*≤ 35 U/l*	*Totals*
Infarction present	925	75	1000
Infarction absent	3075	55925	59000
Totals	4000	56000	60000

The characteristics of the test in this particular situation then can be calculated and are as follows:

$$\text{Prevalence} = \frac{1000}{60000} \times 100 = 1.7\%$$

$$\text{Sensitivity} = \frac{925}{1000} \times 100 = 93\%$$

Specificity $= \dfrac{55925}{59000} \times 100 = 95\%$

Predictive value of a positive test $= \dfrac{925}{4000} \times 100 = 23\%$

Predictive value of a negative test $= \dfrac{55925}{56000} \times 100 = 99\%$

Efficiency $= \dfrac{56850}{60000} \times 100 = 95\%$

This test has a high sensitivity and specificity but the predictive value of a positive test is low compared to the situation where the same test is used only to assess patients admitted to the coronary care unit.

This highlights a further very important point. *Predictive value is directly related to disease prevalence.* As a further example, the effect of prevalence on predictive value for an excellent test with sensitivity and specificity both 95% is shown in Table 7.6.

Table 7.6.

Disease prevalence (%)	Predictive value (%)
0.1	2
1	16
2	28
5	50
10	68
15	77
20	83
25	86
50	95

Two consequences of particular relevance follow from this relationship between predictive value and prevalence. Firstly, because the predictive value improves with disease prevalence, a most important role for the clinician is to raise the prevalence of disease in the population of patients on whom tests are requested by careful assessment of the patients and, using clinical judgement, requesting laboratory tests on only those patients who are considered likely to have disease. Adoption of this strategy, in contrast to the use of tests in profiling or screening modes (*see* Chapter 1), does lead to better test requesting and easier result interpretation. Secondly, this relationship is vital to remember when the published results of assessments of new or existing laboratory tests are being evaluated. Often such work is performed in research laboratories where a common practice is to take equal numbers of patients with disease and of control individuals who do not have disease. The prevalence of disease in this group is 50% and the predictive value of a positive test will appear to be high, as shown in Table 7.7.

Table 7.7.

| | *Prevalence of disease : 50%* | |
Sensitivity %	Specificity %	Predictive value %
70	70	70
80	70	73
80	80	80
90	90	90
90	95	95
95	99	99
99	99	99

Because the predictive value of the test might appear satisfactory and, in all these examples, greater numbers of true positive and negative test results exist than false negative and positive test results, the test is added to the repertoire of the clinical laboratory. However, the disease sought is not common and, in real clinical practice, only 1% of patients on whom the test is performed do actually have the disease. In this situation, with the prevalence at 1%, tests with the same sensitivities and specificities shown in Table 7.7 have markedly lower predictive values (Table 7.8).

Table 7.8.

| | *Prevalence of disease : 1%* | |
Sensitivity %	Specificity %	Predictive value %
70	70	2
80	70	3
80	80	4
90	90	8
90	95	15
95	99	49
99	99	50

This example demonstrates one of the reasons why, as is commonly experienced, a new laboratory test is introduced with great hopes for its potential but the test is found on wider usage over a longer time period to be of little real value in everyday clinical practice.

It is also important to note, from the examples discussed previously using AST in the coronary care unit and on hospitalized patients in general, is that the sensitivity and specificity are not identical in both groups. This is due to the populations in the groups possessing different characteristics. Again when assessing the published literature it is important to remember that the usual practice is to perform a new test on persons who are clearly diseased and on very healthy control subjects. The results obtained in studies designed this way may not reflect the findings seen if the test is subsequently introduced into clinical practice. This is because the test will be applied to patients with minor degrees of disease and equivocal signs and symptoms. Such patients often do not have unequivocal laboratory test results.

7.7 Selection of a test with appropriate characteristics

Bearing in mind that sensitivity is inversely related to specificity and predictive value is directly related to disease prevalence, the characteristics of a laboratory test should be carefully selected in relation to the clinical purposes to which the test is applied.

High sensitivity (no false negative results) is advantageous if the disease is (i) serious and (ii) treatable. Since a test cannot have both 100% sensitivity and specificity, if there are no false negative results then there must be false positive results; this is acceptable if these do not cause harm of any type, because they can be distinguished from true positive results by adoption of some further testing strategy. Examples of diseases for which such a test is required are phaeochromocytoma and phenylketonuria.

High specificity (no false positive results) is advantageous if (i) the disease is serious but not amenable to treatment and (ii) knowledge that the disease is absent has value. As discussed above, if there are no false positive results, there will, of necessity, be false negative results; these are not of great significance, however, because the disease is not treatable and, in most cases, the patient will seek medical attention again. It is more important in this particular situation for all positive results to be true because it would be harmful to label a patient incorrectly as having a serious untreatable disease. The classic example of a disease for which such a test is required is multiple sclerosis.

High efficiency is advantageous if (i) the disease is serious and treatable and (ii) false positive and false negative results are *both* to be avoided as far as possible because the disease is treatable and it is wished to initiate therapy in all cases and because the disease label should not be given unnecessarily since some type of adverse effect will be a consequence. Examples are diabetes mellitus and myocardial infarction.

7.8 The advantage of multiple reference limits

Traditionally, laboratories and clinicians use one reference limit at each boundary between the distributions of results generated on the diseased and the healthy. As has been discussed in detail above, the sensitivity and specificity of a test can be altered simply by changing this reference limit. Moreover, many studies have been shown that clinicians in practice do use different decision limits, these being the levels above (or below) which clinical action is taken (*see* Further reading[3]). A solution to such problems is the adoption of the use of well defined multiple reference limits.

An excellent example of this strategy is that recently advocated by the World Health Organization for use in the assessment of diabetes mellitus (*see* Further reading[4]). Patients are classified on the basis of the results of plasma glucose assays as diabetic, non-diabetic or equivocal. The patients with equivocal results are then further assessed by a dynamic function test, the glucose tolerance test. This approach is shown in Fig. 7.3.

Analytical imprecision, preanalytical variation, biological variation and inaccuracy (*see* earlier chapters) mean that every numerical result does have inherent error. The limits set for definitive action and inaction should take account of this variation and only results which are clearly components of the distributions of the diseased and the healthy should be classified as such. The equivocal group will include patients who are both diseased and healthy but have test results which are not in one of the clear cut groups at least in part due to this

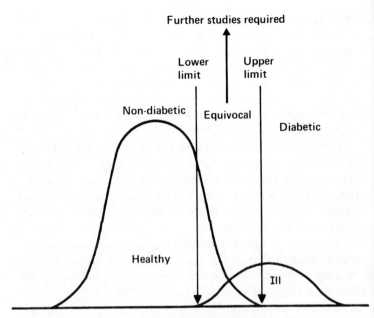

Fig. 7.3. Example of the benefit of using two reference limits to divide the population into three groups; example based upon the World Health Organization recommendations for the assessment of diabetes mellitus.

variation; these patients will likely be classified correctly on further testing.

This approach has much to commend it and is considered more appropriate than use of either a single definitive limit, as is usual practice and seen in some clinical algorithms (*see* Chapter 8) or a single rather vague limit, for example, that advocated as the criteria for initiation of treatment of hyper-cholesterolaemia, that is: detect and treat those and their close relatives with concentrations around and above 8.0 mmol/l (*see* Further reading[2]).

7.9   Multiple testing

It is not usual practice for clinicians to use a single laboratory test in either the investigation or monitoring of patients. The predictive value model can be used in situations where more than one test is used and the text by Galen and Gambino (*see* Further reading[1]) should be consulted for a detailed exposition.

Two tests can be used either sequentially or together. When tests are used sequentially (the series approach), it is usual to cascade positive test results and only carry out the second laboratory test when the result of the first test is positive. In contrast, when two tests are done simultaneously (the parallel approach), the model frequently adopted declares a positive test result when either, or both, of the tests has, or have, positive result(s).

It can be shown that the series testing approach has fewer false positive results than the parallel testing approach but there are more false negative results. In terms of the characteristics of the model, series testing has lower sensitivity and higher specificity than parallel testing.

These comments apply only to two tests which are independent.

7.10   Objective selection of tests

The clinical laboratory selects the tests which form components of its repertoire for a number of reasons which include (i) financial resources, (ii) staff availability and skills, (iii) available instrumentation, (iv) number of tests requested, (v) type of patient on whom specimens are taken, (vi) philosophical approach, particularly of the senior staff, and (viii) demands of particular clinicians. The selection of tests should be more objective and the predictive value model provides a means to judge alternative procedures using the clinical requirements of the test as the major determinant.

For example, many tests have been proposed as the best first line assay for the detection of thyrometabolic disorders. Data available in the laboratory of the author (from Miss M.C.K. Browning) show that, in patients who had been clinically judged and very soundly biochemically classified by a thyroliberin test (TRH test), total thyroxine, free thyroxine and free triiodothyronine had characteristics as shown for *hyperthyroid* patients (Table 7.9). In this study, conventional reference limits were used; this, as alluded to earlier, has some disadvantage.

Table 7.9.

	Total thyroxine	Free thyroxine	Free tri-iodothyronine
Sensitivity (%)	69	100	77
Specificity (%)	90	92	92
Predictive value (%)	75	87	83
Efficiency (%)	91	98	94

Since hyperthyroidism (i) can have serious consequences, (ii) is treatable and (iii) false positive and negative results may both have deleterious consequences, a test with the highest *efficiency* is clearly clinically required. Analysis of the data shows that free thyroxine assay is the most appropriate test in this situation. The same conclusion does apply to tests applied to hypothyroid patients. Thus, the predictive value model gives objective justification for use of this particular clinical laboratory test.

The free thyroxine test has a sensitivity of 100% and therefore will have, and does have, a specificity less than 100%, namely 92%. This means that no cases of hyperthyroidism will be missed but that 8% of persons who do not have hyperthyroidism will be labelled as having a positive test result. In practice, since hyperthyroidism is generally considered to have a prevalence of 0.2%, it is of interest to assess the outcome of testing a large population using this good laboratory procedure and use the predictive value model to help decide on appropriate test strategies.

If all 100 000 patients admitted to hospital during one year were tested, then, since the prevalence of hyperthyroidism is 0.2%, 200 of these patients would have hyperthyroidism.

Testing the 100 000 patients would give the results in Table 7.10, since the sensitivity is 100% and the specificity 92%.

Table 7.10.

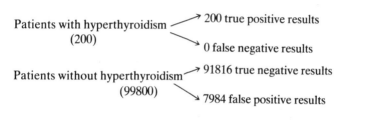

Patients with hyperthyroidism (200) → 200 true positive results
→ 0 false negative results

Patients without hyperthyroidism (99800) → 91816 true negative results
→ 7984 false positive results

Thus, the yield of positive results is 8184 but the predictive value of the positive result is only 2.4%. This situation can be handled using a number of strategies which can all be logically examined using the predictive value model principles discussed in detail in this chapter.

Firstly, since predictive value is directly proportional to disease prevalence, if clinicians carefully assessed the patients and only performed the test on the 3% (say) admitted with some signs and symptoms of hyperthyroidism, then only 3000 would be tested, all 200 with hyperthyroidism detected (100% sensitivity) and only 224 false positive results would be generated.

Secondly, the *same* test could be *repeated* on all 8184 patients with a positive result. The 200 patients with hyperthyroidism would all have a second positive result since the test has 100% sensitivity. If the 7984 patients without hyperthyroidism who had an initial false positive test result did redistribute themselves throughout the distribution seen for all patients who did not have thyroid disease, then 639 (8%) of the 7984 would have a second positive test; these test results, of course, would still be false positive results. A further repeat test on these patients who now had positive test results (200 true and 639 false) would result in only 51 of the 251 positive results found being false positive results. This repetitive procedure using the same test is shown diagramatically in Fig. 7.4.

Thirdly, a second different test could be applied to all patients with a positive test result in sequential cascading approach. This second test could be (i) a similar test, for example, total or free triiodothyronine, (ii) a rather different test, for example, thyrotrophin (TSH), (iii) a dynamic function test, for example, the thyroliberin (TRH) test or (iv) a procedure outside the remit of the clinical laboratory. The ideal is a test with 100% specificity and a high sensitivity such as the newer methods for TSH assay which have very low detection limits. If the sensitivity of such a test was 98% (2% false negative results), then application of this to the 8184 positive test results (200 true positive and 7984 false positive results) would clearly label all 7984 patients without disease as healthy and only 4 of the hyperthyroid patients would, on the basis of this test, have negative test results.

The strategy which should be adopted will depend on a number of local circumstances but, in any case, should be determined as objectively as possible.

7.11   Further approaches

One of the uses of the predictive value model is to compare the utility of clinical laboratory tests. A more detailed comparison than that available by the simple model is obtained by use of *receiver operating characteristic (ROC) curves*. These are

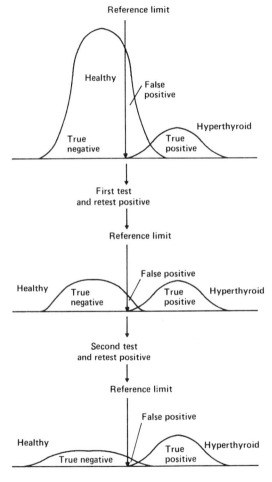

Fig. 7.4. Replicate testing of a population when the test has 100% sensitivity.

becoming more frequently used in the clinical literature. A plot is prepared of the true positive rate against the false positive rate, that is,

$$\frac{TP}{TP+FN}(\text{sensitivity}) \text{ is plotted against } \frac{FP}{FP+TN}(\text{100-specificity})$$

A model ROC curve is shown in Fig. 7.5. The advantage of the use of these curves is that they allow comparison of tests without selection of any particular upper (or lower) reference limit or any particular sensitivity or specificity. Each limit has, as a single point on the ROC curve, a true positive and matching false positive rate. The appropriate use of ROC curves is discussed by Zweig and Robertson (*see* Further reading[5]).

A further derived quantity is the *likelihood ratio*; this can be calculated for either detection or exclusion of disease.
The likelihood ratio for detection is:

$$\frac{TP}{FP} = \frac{\text{sensitivity}}{\text{100-specificity}}$$

The likelihood ratio for exclusion is:

$$\frac{FN}{TN} = \frac{\text{100-sensitivity}}{\text{specificity}}$$

These derived ratios are not currently widely used in clinical or laboratory practice.

7.12 Summary

The predictive value model is simple to apply to both single and multiple laboratory tests. The model has a multiplicity of uses including (i) the determination of the true meaning of positive and negative test results, (ii) the assessment of the most appropriate test for a specific clinical purpose and (iii)

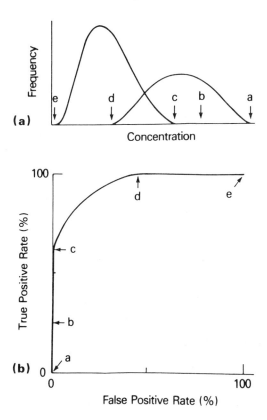

Fig. 7.5. (a) Hypothetical frequency distribution, with left-hand curve representing results from healthy individuals and right-hand curve representing results from diseased individuals. (b) Receiver operating characteristic curve (corresponding to data in (a)), generated by varying the reference and then plotting the resulting pairs of true- and false-positive rates. a–e mark points corresponding to reference limits in upper panel. The curve from c to d describes the test's performance in the crucial overlap region. From Zweig M.H. & Robertson E.A. (1982) *Clinical Chemistry,* **28,** 1275 (with permission).

the selection of the best strategy for investigation of patients with particular diseases.

An excellent use of the model is the objective evaluation of previously published data and logical extension of the experimental data contained in such papers to everyday practice.

The model, however, is not without drawbacks. The true definition of disease and health may be very difficult. Sensitivity and specificity are dependent on the reference limit used and it may be difficult to extrapolate data presented in the usual format to other reference limits. The repetitive testing model assumes that redistribution of a component of the population occurs throughout the distribution of the original population when retesting is undertaken; biological variation data (*see* Chapter 6) would suggest that this does not really occur in most cases.

A number of further approaches are possible; the use of receiver operating characteristic curves has advantages in comparison of the utility of different tests.

Further reading

1   Galen R.S. & Gambino S.R. (1975) *Beyond Normality: the Predictive Value and Efficiency of Medical Diagnoses.* John Wiley and Sons, New York.
2   Oliver M.F. (1984) Why measure cholesterol after myocardial infarction, and when? *British Medical Journal,* **289,** 161.
3   Skendzel L.P., Barnett R.N. & Platt R. (1985) Medically useful criteria for analytic performance of laboratory tests. *American Journal of Clinical Pathology,* **83,** 200.
4   World Health Organization (1980) *WHO Expert Committee on Diabetes Mellitus. Second Report. Technical Report Series 646.* WHO, Geneva.
5   Zweig M.H. & Robertson E.A. (1982) Why we need better test evaluations. *Clinical Chemistry,* **28,** 1272.

Chapter 8
The Unexpected Test Result

8.1 Introduction

In this text, those aspects of clinical laboratory tests which pose real or potential difficulties have been discussed in detail.

In most clinical situations, it is hoped that the correct specimen will be appropriately collected from a well documented properly prepared patient and this specimen will be transported timeously to the clinical laboratory along with a completed request form detailing all of the information required by both the clinical laboratory and the clinician for the correct interpretation of the result, namely:

(i)   unambiguous patient identification, for example, patient name and unit number,

(ii)   age and sex of patient,

(iii)   name of requesting clinician,

(iv)   source of request, for example, hospital, ward, clinic,

(v)   specimen type; blood, serum, plasma, urine, cerebrospinal fluid, faeces, other fluid,

(vi)   date and time of specimen collection, duration of collection period if timed, or timing of samples during dynamic function tests,

(vii)   clinical problem of patient and reason for request,

(viii)   drug or intravenous therapy, and

(ix)   posture of patient at specimen collection; ambulent, sitting or recumbent.

The specimen will be appropriately documented and handled, analyses of acceptable performance characteristics will be performed with adequate quality control procedures monitoring analytical standards and numerical results will be returned complete with appropriate reference intervals. The

161

results will then be interpreted for the individual patient with background knowledge of the clinical sensitivity, specificity and predictive value of the test in the particular clinical situation and, finally, appropriate clinical action will be taken.

In some instances, however, the numerical result will be difficult to interpret or will be unexpected.

The unexpected clinical laboratory test result, that is the result that does not fit in with the clinical picture, does cause much concern and strategies to deal with this situation are addressed in this final chapter, in large part in order to review the entire content of this text.

8.2 Strategies to deal with the unexpected result

The strategies often adopted to deal with the unexpected result are (i) simply to ignore it or (ii) to label the result as a laboratory error or a blunder (defined as a stupid and careless mistake) and disregard it. There is no doubt that blunders are made with regard to all of the following:

(i)   patient identification,
(ii)   specimen collection,
(iii)   specimen labelling,
(iv)   transport and handling,
(v)   laboratory specimen identification,
(vi)   analytical procedure,
(vii)   calculation of result from raw data,
(viii) recording of result and
(ix)   insertion of result on to a report.

However, rather than the clinician merely disregarding the unexpected result or the perpetrator of the event attempting to cover up a known blunder, other strategies should be adopted. It is particularly important for clinical laboratory staff to inform clinicians about obvious blunders made in the ward or clinic and for clinicians to notify clinical laboratory staff concerning other blunders so that educational and/or quality control measures can be initiated in order to attempt to eliminate similar mistakes in the future.

A careful search for results of the same tests performed earlier on the patient should be initiated and objective comparison of results undertaken, bearing in mind the considerations detailed in Chapter 6.

The follow-up of the unexpected result of the type where the result that appears to be outside reference values may be assisted by the use of algorithms (*see* Further reading[1]). This

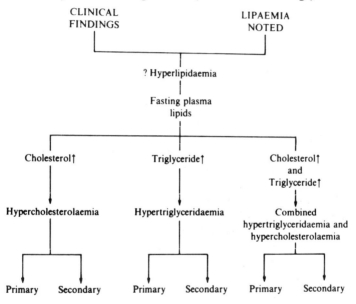

RR: Plasma (fasting) cholesterol 3.5–7.3 mmol/l
triglyceride 0.3–1.7 mmol/l

N.B. Fasting requires 12–16 h without food.

Fig. 8.1. Algorithm to aid in the interpretation of results showing hyperlipidaemia. From Walmsley R.N. and White G.H. (1985) *Pocket Diagnostic Clinical Chemistry*, p. 139. Blackwell Scientific Publications Limited, Melbourne.

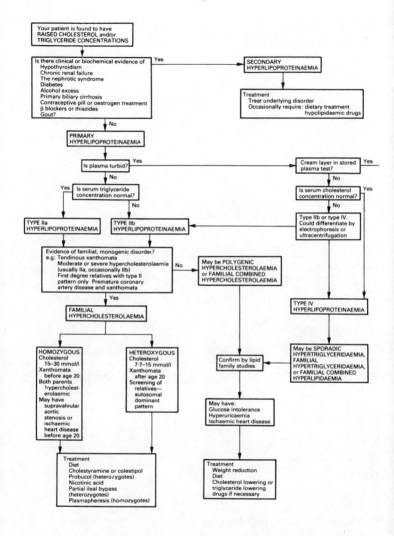

Your patient is found to have RAISED CHOLESTEROL and/or TRIGLYCERIDE CONCENTRATIONS

Is there clinical or biochemical evidence of
Hypothyroidism
Chronic renal failure
The nephrotic syndrome
Diabetes
Alcohol excess
Primary biliary cirrhosis
Contraceptive pill or oestrogen treatment
β blockers or thiazides
Gout? — Yes → SECONDARY HYPERLIPOPROTEINAEMIA

Treatment
Treat underlying disorder
Occasionally require: dietary treatment
hypolipidaemic drugs

No ↓

PRIMARY HYPERLIPOPROTEINAEMIA

Is plasma turbid? — Yes → Cream layer in stored plasma test? — Yes →

No ↓   No ↓

Is serum triglyceride concentration normal? — Yes

Is serum cholesterol concentration normal? — Yes →

No ↓

TYPE IIa HYPERLIPOPROTEINAEMIA   TYPE IIb HYPERLIPOPROTEINAEMIA

Type IIb or type IV. Could differentiate by electrophoresis or ultracentrifugation

Evidence of familial, monogenic disorder?
e.g: Tendinous xanthomata
Moderate or severe hypercholesterolaemia (usually IIa, occasionally IIb)
First degree relatives with type II pattern only Premature coronary artery disease and xanthomata — No → May be POLYGENIC HYPERCHOLESTEROLAEMIA or FAMILIAL COMBINED HYPERCHOLESTEROLAEMIA

Yes ↓

FAMILIAL HYPERCHOLESTEROLAEMIA

TYPE IV HYPERLIPOPROTEINAEMIA

HOMOZYGOUS
Cholesterol 15–30 mmol/l
Xanthomata before age 20
Both parents hypercholesterolaemic
May have supravalvular aortic stenosis or ischaemic heart disease before age 20

HETEROXYGOUS
Cholesterol 7·7–15 mmol/l
Xanthomata after age 20
Screening of relatives—autosomal dominant pattern

May be SPORADIC HYPERTRIGLYCERIDAEMIA, FAMILIAL HYPERTRIGLYCERIDAEMIA, or FAMILIAL COMBINED HYPERLIPIDAEMIA

Confirm by lipid family studies

May have:
Glucose intolerance
Hyperuricaemia
Ischaemic heart disease

Treatment
Diet
Cholestyramine or colestipol
Probucol (heterozygotes)
Nicotinic acid
Partial ileal bypass (heterozygotes)
Plasmapheresis (homozygotes)

Treatment
Weight reduction
Diet
Cholesterol lowering or triglyceride lowering drugs if necessary

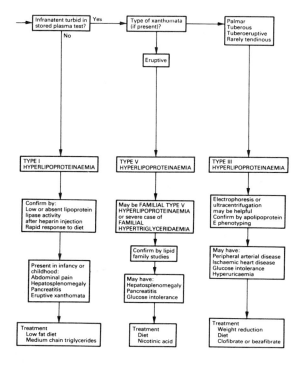

Fig. 8.2. Algorithm to aid in the interpretation of results showing hyperlipidaemia. From Murchison L.E. (1985) *British Medical Journal*, **290**, 536 (with permission).

approach is becoming utilized more and more in the literature, both in all types of texts and in medical journals. Algorithms can be defined as sequences of logical steps which carry out specific tasks, operations and transformation of data, or as exact descriptions of solutions to problems. They are usually displayed in flow charts which show the processes involved in making decisions. Because they often depict branching logic, the flow charts are sometimes called decision trees. Two published algorithms dealing with hyperlipidaemia are shown in Figs. 8.1 and 8.2 (*see* Further reading[2,3]). The first algorithm has perhaps some use in education and as an *aide-mémoire* for students to follow in order to aid in the interpretation of an unusual result. The second algorithm is more useful in following up the unexpected result but has the disadvantages of all algorithms of this type in that (i) the criteria for 'normality' and 'abnormality' are not well defined, (ii) the possibilities of errors, blunders and preanalytical sources of variation are not considered, (iii) good clinical skills and judgements make strict adherance to the algorith unnecessary and wasteful in many situations and (iv) not every patient will fit in exactly with the algorithm.

It is considered that *before* the unexpected result is followed up using such approaches, it is necessary to consider all of the points discussed in this text. The checklist shown in Table 8.1 may assist this process.

Table 8.1. Checklist to aid in the assessment of the unexpected result before initiation of clinical action.

Preanalysis	Food and drink intake
	Alcohol intake
	Posture
	Stress
	Pregnancy
	Exercise
	Hospitalization

Drug therapy
Previous medical and/or surgical
  care
Effects of other constituents
  present

Specimen collection	Patient identification
	Blood collection site
	Contamination of specimen
	Appropriate anticoagulation
	Haemolysis
	Tourniquet application
	Urine collection completeness
	Contamination of urine
	Appropriate preservative and/or stabilizer
	Cerebrospinal fluid contamination
	Adequate transport
	Correct storage
	Separation of plasma

Laboratory factors	Specimen mix-up
	Analytical error
	Calculation error
	Recording of result

Reference values	Appropriate interval available
	Dependence on
	age body mass
	sex other factors

Biological variation	Specimen collected at correct time
	Existence of daily, monthly or seasonal rhythm

Predictive value	Appropriateness of test chosen
	Results in the ill (sensitivity)
	Results in the healthy (specificity)
	Meaning of a positive test
	Strategy for further testing

In any case, before any unexpected result is acted upon, it is good practice to repeat carefully the clinical laboratory test under optimal conditions.

Further reading

1   Lundberg G.D. Ed. (1983) *Using the Clinical Laboratory in Medical Decision Making.* American Society of Clinical Pathologists, Chicago.
2   Murchison L.E. (1985) Hyperlipidaemia. *British Medical Journal,* **290,** 536.
3   Walmsley R.N. & White G.H. (1985) *Pocket Diagnostic Clinical Chemistry.* Blackwell Scientific Publications Ltd., Melbourne.

Index